Regenerative Medicine

Edited by Mahmood S Choudhery

Published in London, United Kingdom

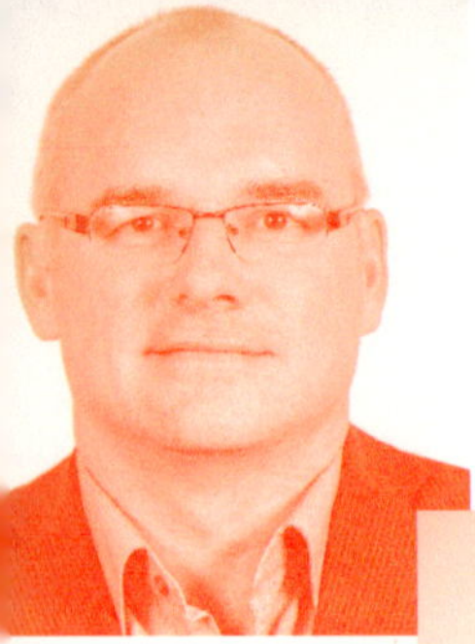
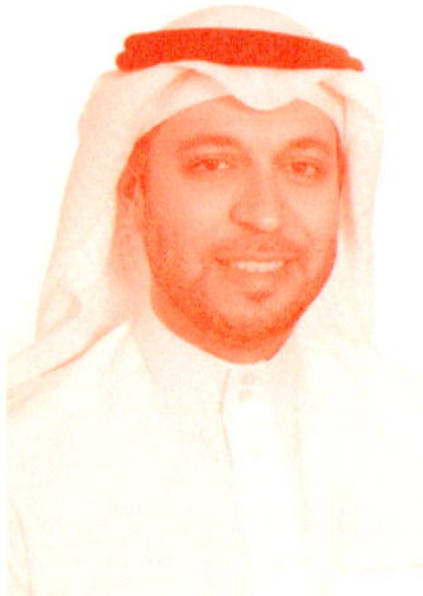
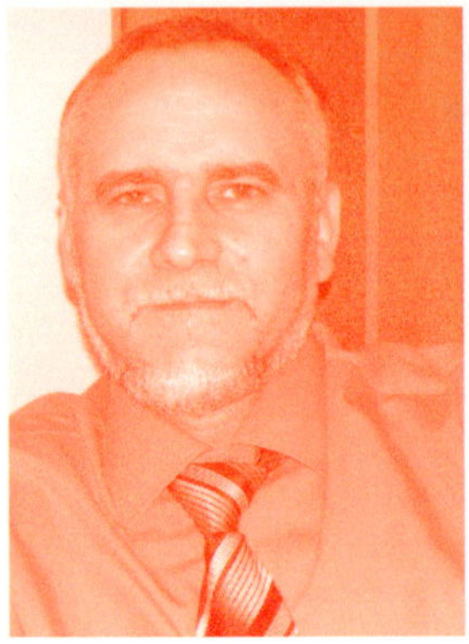
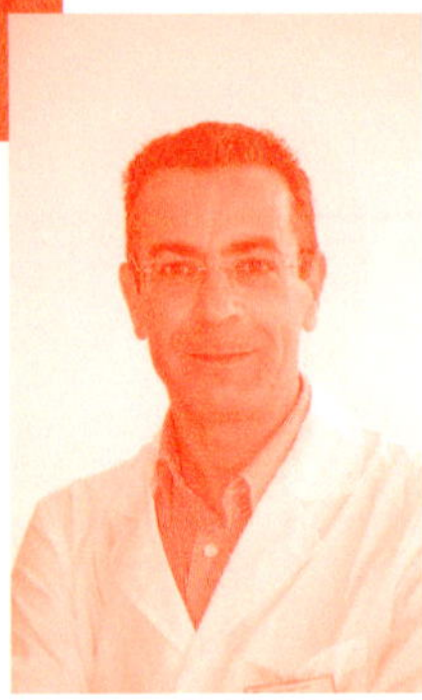
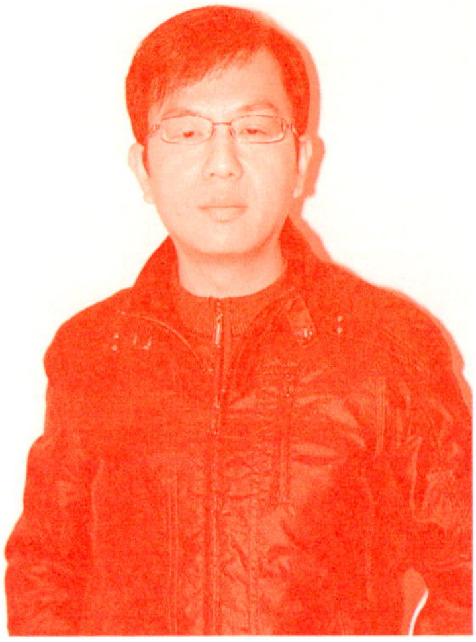
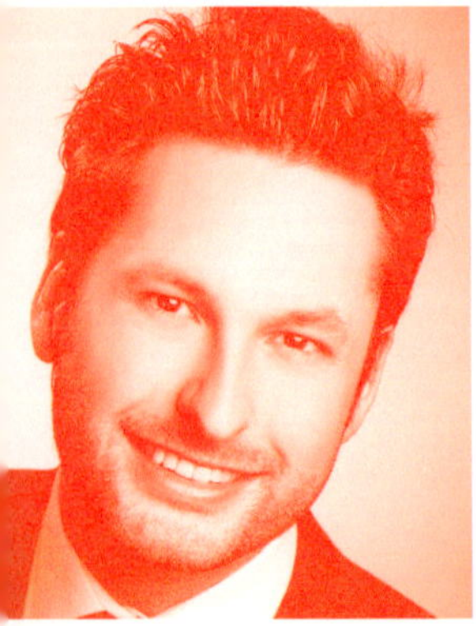
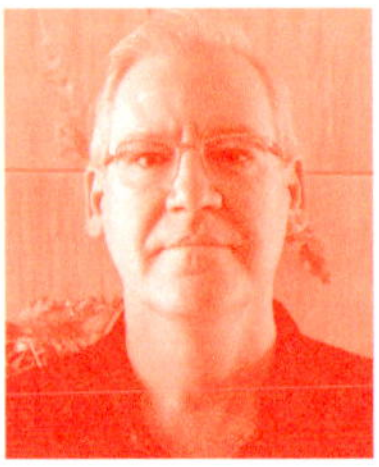

IntechOpen

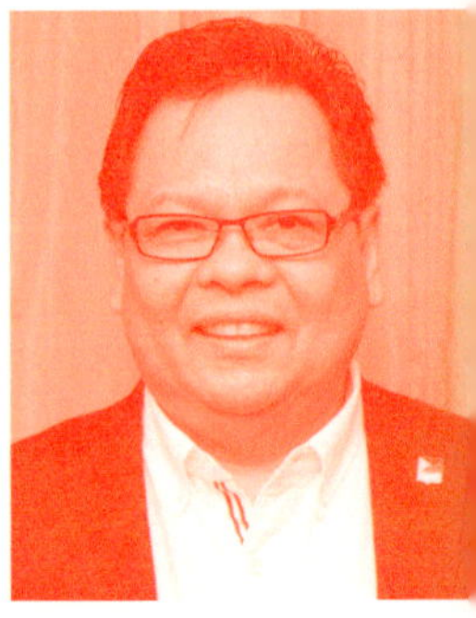
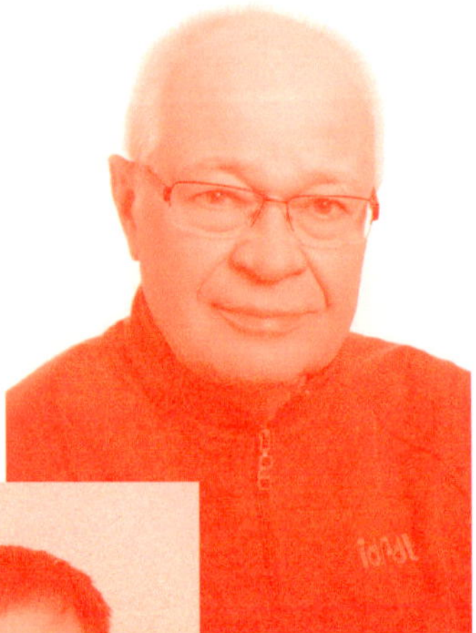
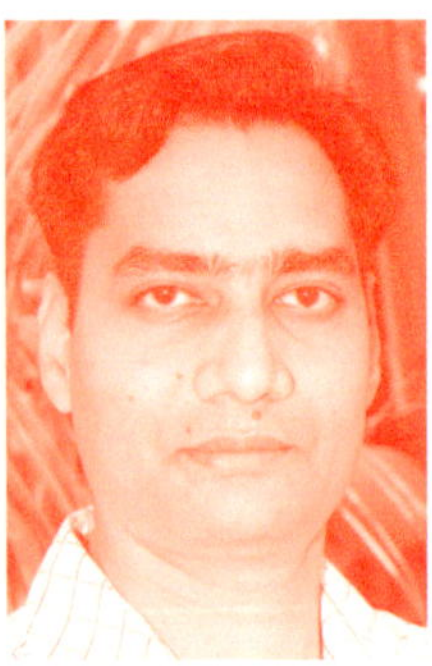
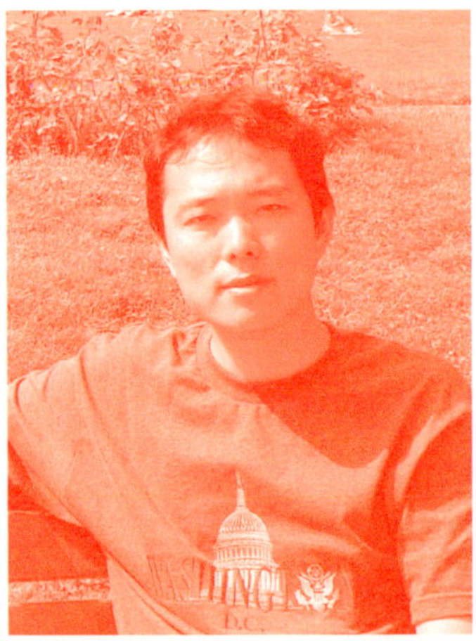
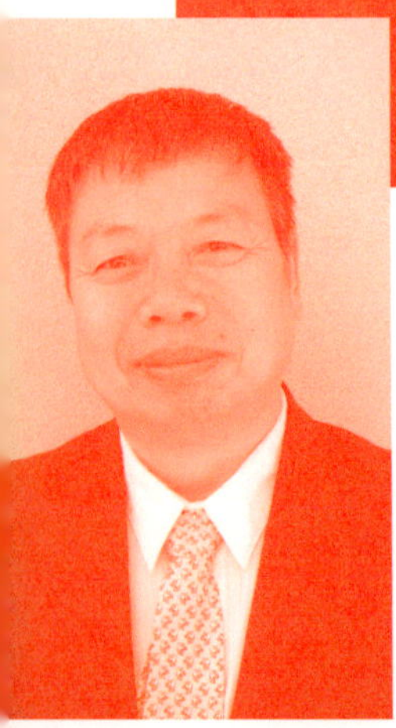
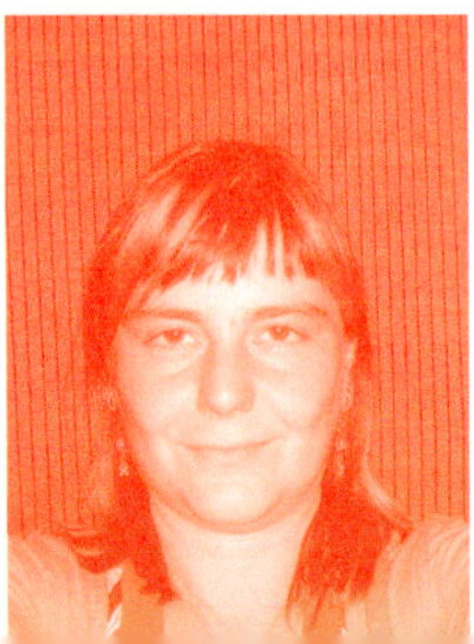

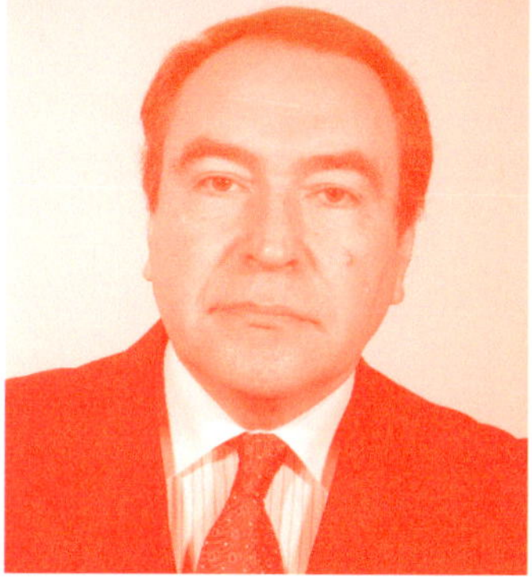
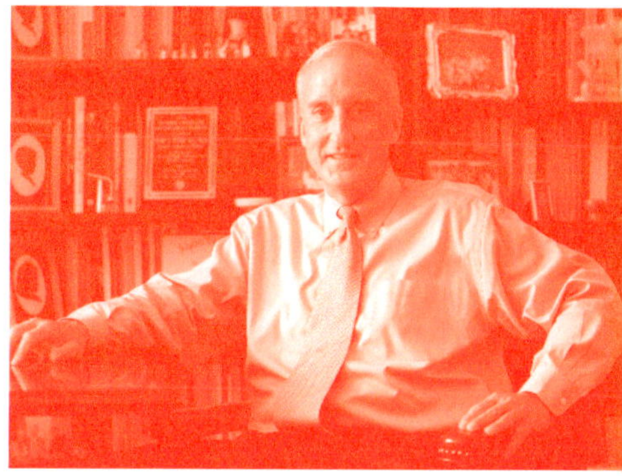
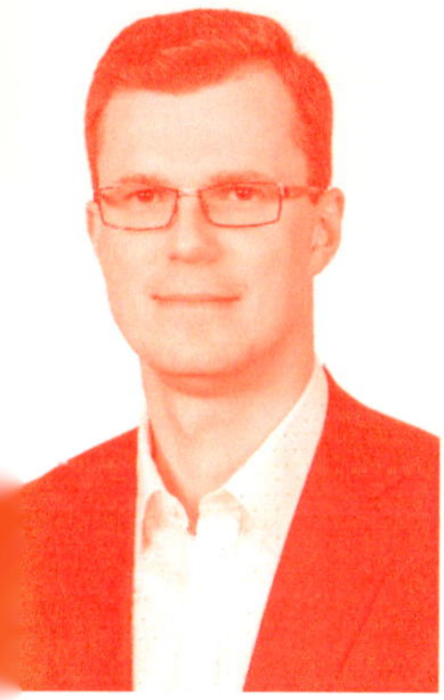
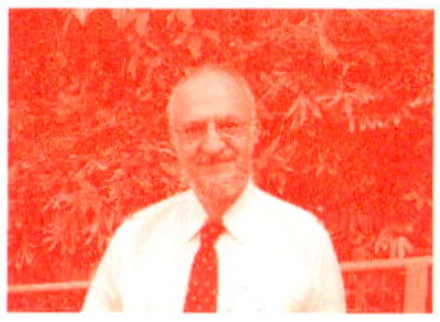
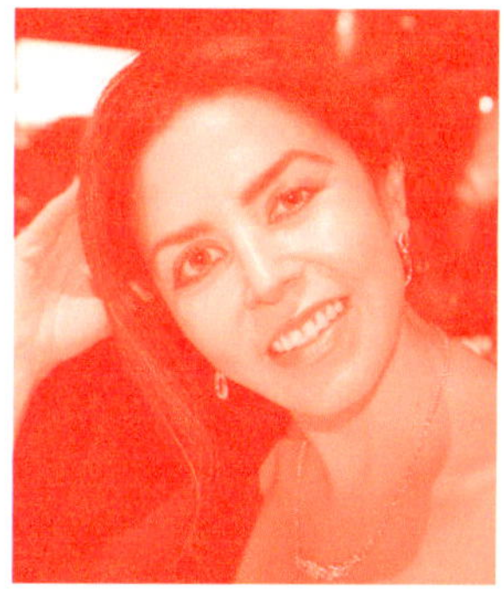

Supporting open minds since 2005

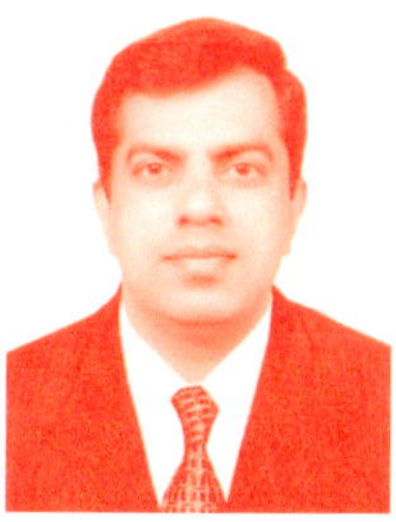
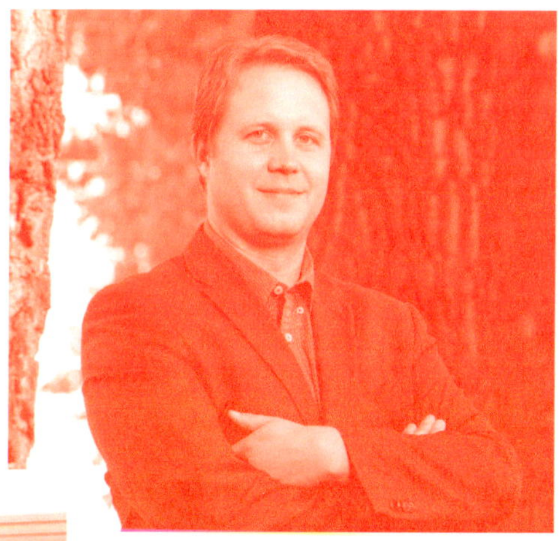
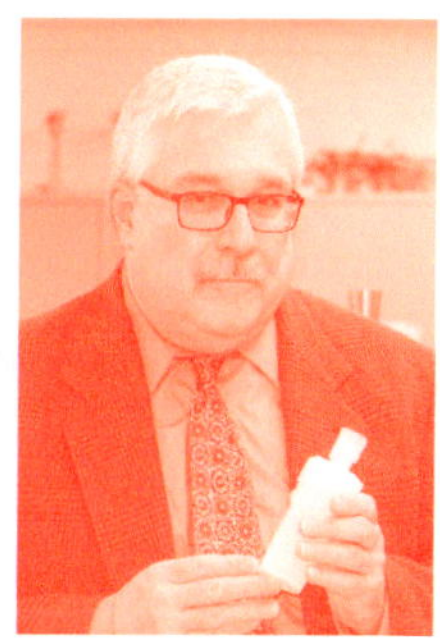
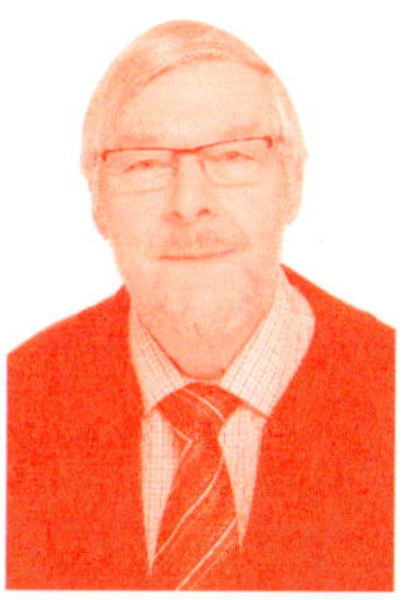
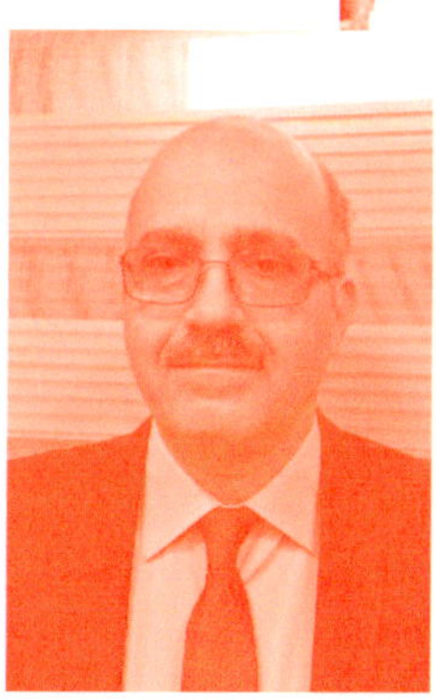
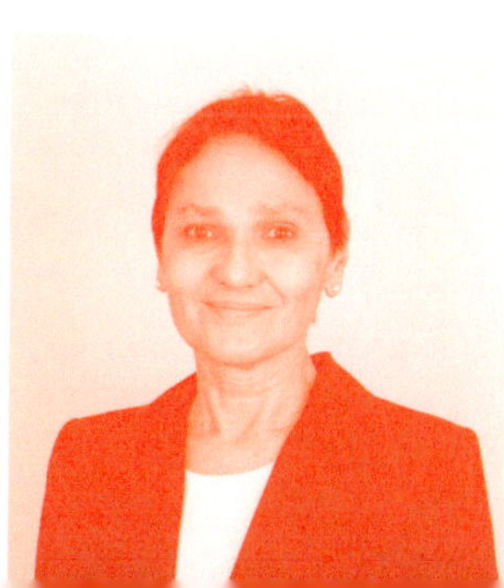
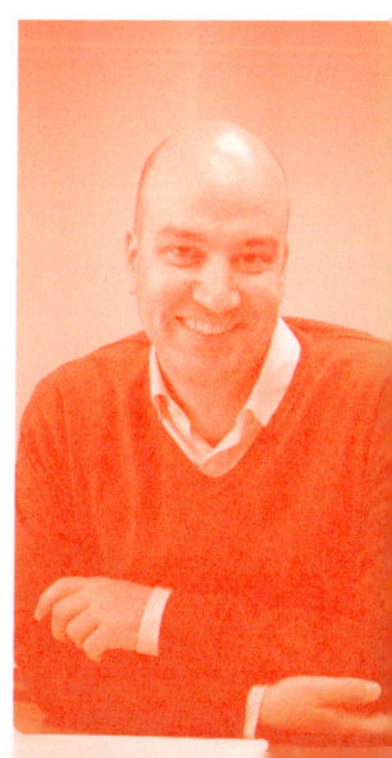

Regenerative Medicine
http://dx.doi.org/10.5772/intechopen.78082
Edited by Mahmood S Choudhery

Contributors
Peter A. Everts, Glenn Flanagan II, Joshua Rothenberg, Kenneth Mautner, Enzo Maria Vingolo, Laura Contento, Antonio Florido, Filippo Avogaro, Paolo Giuseppe Limoli, Loubna Mazini, Mikel Sánchez, Maider Beitia, Orlando Pompei, Cristina Jorquera, Pello Sánchez, Jorge Knörr, Francisco Soldado, Leonor López, Jaime Oraa, Ane Miren Bilbao, Nicolás Fiz, Jorge Guadilla, Beatriz Aizpurua, Juan Azofra, Diego Delgado, Bushra Bashir, Mehmood-S Choudhery, Ick Soo Kim, Davood Kharaghani, Zahra Tajbakhsh, Phan Duy Nam, Luc Rochette, Gabriel Malka, Ijaz Hussain

First published in London, United Kingdom, 2020 by IntechOpen
IntechOpen is the global imprint of INTECHOPEN LIMITED, registered in England and Wales, registration number: 11086078, 5 Princes Gate Court, London, SW7 2QJ, United Kingdom
Printed in Croatia

British Library Cataloguing-in-Publication Data
A catalogue record for this book is available from the British Library

Additional hard and PDF copies can be obtained from orders@intechopen.com

Regenerative Medicine
Edited by Mahmood S Choudhery
p. cm.
Print ISBN 978-1-83881-927-9
Online ISBN 978-1-83881-928-6
eBook (PDF) ISBN 978-1-83881-929-3

For EU product safety concerns:
IN TECH d.o.o., Prolaz Marije Krucifikse Kozulić 3, 51000 Rijeka, Croatia, info@intechopen.com or visit our website at intechopen.com.

Meet the editor

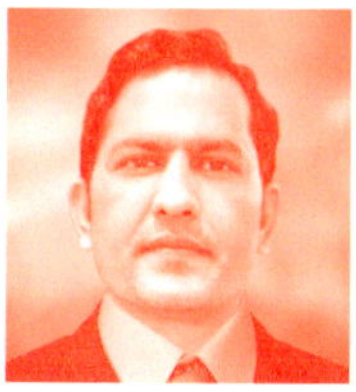

Dr. Mahmood S. Choudhery is Associate Professor of Biomedical Sciences, working at the Tissue Engineering and Regenerative Medicine Laboratory of the Department of Biomedical Sciences at King Edward Medical University. He received his BSc (Hons) from Punjab University and worked for his PhD at the National Center of Excellence in Molecular Biology (CEMB), Punjab University, and the University of Arizona, USA. He continued his research on stem cells at the University of Arizona in the Dr. David T. Harris Laboratory. At King Edward Medical University, along with teaching, Dr. Choudhery researches stem cell-based regenerative therapies. Dr. Choudhery is an editorial board member of several international journals of high repute and has published his research work in many leading journals.

Dedication

To my Daughter, Hafsa, and my sons, Kashan and Affan. You are my love and the center of my world. To my mother and father who are the "wind beneath my wings."

Contents

Preface XI

Chapter 1 1
The Rationale of Autologously Prepared Bone Marrow Aspirate Concentrate for use in Regenerative Medicine Applications
by Peter A. Everts, Glenn Flanagan II, Joshua Rothenberg and Kenneth Mautner

Chapter 2 41
Adipose-Derived Stem Cells (ADSCs) and Growth Differentiation Factor 11 (GDF11): Regenerative and Antiaging Capacity for the Skin
by Loubna Mazini, Luc Rochette and Gabriel Malka

Chapter 3 67
Isolation, Activation, and Mechanism of Action of Platelet-Rich Plasma and Its Applications for Joint Repair
by Mikel Sánchez, Maider Beitia, Orlando Pompei, Cristina Jorquera, Pello Sánchez, Jorge Knörr, Francisco Soldado, Leonor López, Jaime Oraa, Ane Miren Bilbao, Nicolás Fiz, Jorge Guadilla, Beatriz Aizpurua, Juan Azofra and Diego Delgado

Chapter 4 93
Regenerative Medicine and Eye Diseases
by Enzo Maria Vingolo, Laura Contento, Antonio Florido, Filippo Avogaro and Paolo Giuseppe Limoli

Chapter 5 119
Application of Nanowires for Retinal Regeneration
by Davood Kharaghani, Zahra Tajbakhsh, Phan Duy Nam and Ick Soo Kim

Chapter 6 137
Hypoxic Preconditioning as a Strategy to Maintain the Regenerative Potential of Mesenchymal Stem Cells
by Bushra Bashir, Mahmood S. Choudhery and Ijaz Hussain

Preface

Regenerative medicine is a promising interdisciplinary field that applies basic principles of engineering and life sciences to repair, replace, or regenerate damaged or lost tissues and organs. Unlike conventional medicine, regenerative medicine uses human cells and other substances to regrow tissues or restore their functions. An important characteristic of regenerative medicine is that its effects, if not permanent, are long lasting. The main aim of regenerative medicine is to use culturing methods to develop techniques and products using the body's own cells for medical treatment. Regenerative medicine combines approaches such as the use of cell-based, cell-free soluble molecules, stem cells from different sources, gene therapy, tissue engineering, reprogramming of cells and, more recently, cell-free regenerative therapies. This book, *Regenerative Medicine*, provides details of recent advancements in regenerative therapies for regenerative medicine applications.

Regenerative medicine therapies have gained significant popularity in recent years and have provided novel therapeutic approaches for a number of diseases. This book examines research in bone marrow aspirates, adipose tissue-derived stem cells and growth differentiation factor 11, platelet-rich plasma, and nanowires for use in regenerative medicine applications. Chapters focus on the use of stem cells (specifically mesenchymal stem cells derived from bone marrow or adipose tissue) and platelet-rich plasma for regenerative purposes. In addition, the book discusses regenerative medicine applications for eyes, skin, musculoskeletal disorders, spinal disorders, critical limb ischemia, and joint degeneration. Further, it covers the role of hypoxic preconditioning as a strategy to enhance the regenerative potential of stem cells. The chapter by Dr. Everts et al., "The Rationale and Roles of Autologous Prepared Bone Marrow Aspirate Concentrate Cells in Regenerative Medicine Applications," highlights the applications of autologous bone marrow-derived concentrate in regenerative medicine. This chapter begins with a brief introduction of stem cells and their different types and addresses the cellular contents of bone marrow tissue, harvesting, and preparation techniques. In addition, this chapter further discusses characteristics of bone marrow-derived mesenchymal stem cells and their applications in musculoskeletal disorders, spinal disorders, chronic wounds, and critical limb ischemia.

The chapter "Adipose-Derived Stem Cells (ADSCs) and Growth Differentiation Factor 11 (GDF11): Regenerative and Antiaging Capacity for the Skin" by Dr. Mazini et al. describes how ADSCs cross-react with GDF11 to assure dermal fibroblasts' and keratinocytes' proliferation to reverse the aging process. It also discusses the involvement of cell signaling pathways related to GDF11 and TGF-β in balancing cell rejuvenation and cell regeneration as well as skin anatomy, mechanism of skin aging, role of ADSCs in skin rejuvenation, and interactions of ASDCs with TFG-β and GDF11 for skin regeneration. Finally, the chapter presents immunomodulatory effects and antiaging mechanisms of ADSCs with respect to TFG- β and GDF11.

"Isolation, Activation and Mechanism of Action of Platelet-Rich Plasma and its Applications for Joint Repair" by Dr. Sanchez et al. highlights the importance of platelet-rich plasma (PRP) use for joint repair. This chapter describes joint physiology and the process of joint degeneration followed by a description of PRP as a bioactive source. It also discusses in detail methods of PRP isolation and preparation, its types, and process of activation. Finally, the chapter describes the therapeutic potential of PRP in joint degeneration and its clinical translation.

In "Regenerative Medicine and Eye Diseases," Dr. Vingolo et al. examine the use of stem cells in ophthalmological pathologies affecting both the anterior and posterior eye segments. The authors review the most relevant clinical trials describing the role and potential of stem cell-based regenerative therapy in corneal and retinal pathology. They also analyze and comment on the results of scientific literature and possible side effects related to the use of stem cell therapy. Further, the chapter describes the route of cell administration and role of regenerative medicine in the anterior and posterior segments of the eye. Finally, the authors share their experience of cell therapy in atrophic retinal diseases.

"Applications of Nanowires for Retinal Diseases" by Dr. Kharaghani et al. provides an introduction of retinal anatomy, retinal disorders, and the latest progress in the research for retinal regeneration and vision using nanowires. In addition, the chapter examines different structures including core-shell and functionalized nanowires with nanoparticles. It also describes the nanowire-based mechanism of retinal regeneration along with challenges and prospects of its use.

In the final chapter, "Hypoxic Preconditioning as a Strategy to Maintain the Regenerative Potential of Mesenchymal Stem Cells," Dr. Bashir et al. discuss hypoxic preconditioning for improving regenerative potential of stem cells. In this chapter, the authors describe how regenerative potential of stem cells is compromised by age of donor and in vitro passaging, and how hypoxic preconditioning could be employed to enhance the age- and passage-depleted function of stem cells.

Although my name appears on this book's cover, I am grateful to the wonderful work of all the authors who contributed chapters. I am also grateful for the support provided by the staff at IntechOpen. I would like to thank my brother Muhammad Hanif for his continuous support and my wife Ruhma Mahmood Choudhery for her assistance and support. Thanks to all my students at King Edward Medical University and those who worked with me at University of Arizona, USA. Thanks also to Professor David T. Harris for his sincere advice and belief in me.

Dr. Mahmood S. Choudhery, PhD
King Edward Medical University,
Lahore, Pakistan

Chapter 1

The Rationale of Autologously Prepared Bone Marrow Aspirate Concentrate for use in Regenerative Medicine Applications

Peter A. Everts, Glenn Flanagan II, Joshua Rothenberg and Kenneth Mautner

Abstract

Autologously prepared bone marrow aspirate concentrates, have the potential to play an adjunctive role in various patient pathologies that have not been able to heal with conventional treatment modalities. The use of bone marrow aspirate (BMA) and concentrates in regenerative medicine treatment plans and clinical applications is based on the fact that bone marrow cells, including progenitor and nucleated cells, platelets, and other cytokines, support in tissue healing and tissue regenerative processes. The use of concentrated BMA cells focuses primarily on mesenchymal stem cells (MSCs), with the ability to self-renew and differentiate into multiple cell types. Concentrated bone marrow cells can be retrieved from harvested BMA and ensuing minimal manipulative cell processing techniques, executed at point of care (POC). The application of bone marrow biological therapies may offer solutions in musculoskeletal pathologies, spinal disorders, chronic wound care, and critical limb ischemia (CLI), to effectively change the local microenvironment to support in tissue healing and facilitate tissue regeneration. This chapter will address the cellular content of bone marrow tissue, harvesting and preparation techniques, and discuss the biological characteristics of individual marrow cells, their inter-connectivity, and deliberate on the effects of BMA concentration.

Keywords: regenerative medicine, bone marrow aspiration, niche microenvironment, bone marrow concentrate, centrifugation, hematopoietic stem cells, mesenchymal stem cells, differentiation, immunomodulation

1. Introduction

The objectives of regenerative medicine applications are to support the body to form new functional tissues to replace degenerative or defective ones and to provide therapeutic treatment for conditions where conventional therapies are inadequate. The human body has an endogenous system of regeneration through stem cells,

IntechOpen

as they are found almost in every type of tissue. Regenerative medicine treatment options using autologous stem cells can be safely executed by well-trained physicians at point of care (POC). This review is not meant to be exhaustive, but our aims are to shed light on the bone marrow progenitor and stem cell mechanisms and highlight present and future applications of autologous bone marrow-derived stem cells in this exciting new regenerative medicine discipline.

In this chapter a definition is provided on embryotic and non-embryotic stem cells, followed by an intensive review of non-embryotic autologous adult stem cells. The use of allogeneic MSCs, the fabrication of engineered constructs by seeding of natural or synthetic scaffolds with cells, released from autologous tissues will not be presented in this chapter, as only relatively few of these cell-based approaches have entered the clinical arena. In particular, we deliberate on the biology and clinical application of mesenchymal stem cells originating from freshly harvested bone marrow. We portray on the techniques of a marrow harvesting procedure using ultrasound and fluoroscopic techniques. Explicit scientific information is provided on the bone marrow aspirate cellular content, their specific biological functions and intercellular interactions, as these, among others, contribute to tissue regeneration following clinical regenerative medicine applications. Furthermore, we underline the differences between bone marrow aspirate and, centrifugated, bone marrow aspirate concentrate injectates, both prepared at point of care from freshly aspirated marrow.

Finally, a condensed literature review addressing a variety of clinical orthobiological indications, spinal disorders, chronic wounds, and critical limb ischemia is provided. Regenerative medicine technologies, using marrow-derived mesenchymal stem cell-based therapies, as part of the regenerative medicine treatment armamentarium, offer solutions to a number of undeniable clinical conditions that have not been able to adequately result in a solution through the use of medicines or surgeries.

2. What are stem cells?

Becker, McCulloch, and Till first conducted experiments that lead to the discovery of stem cells in 1963. After injecting bone marrow cells into irradiated mice, nodules developed in proportion to the number of bone marrow cells injected, and they concluded that each nodule arose from a single marrow cell. At a later stage, they produced evidence that these cells were capable of endless self-renewal, which is as we know now, a fundamental feature of stem cells [1]. A stem cell is a type of cell that is non-specific/specialized in its function; in contrast, for instance, a heart or brain cell is functionally specific.

Generally, we recognize two types of stem cells, embryonic and non-embryonic, with two defining properties. Firstly, they have the capacity of self-renewal, therefore giving rise to more stem cells. Secondly, they are capable of differentiating into different lineages under appropriate conditions.

Embryonic stem cells (ESCs) are obtained from 5- to 12-day-old embryos, and they are pluripotent and have a high plasticity as they can differentiate into ectoderm, mesoderm, and endoderm layers, whereas non-embryonic stem cells (non-ESCs) are multipotent, and it appears that they are able to form multiple cell lineages which form an entire tissue, usually specific to one germ layer, e.g., adult stem cells [2].

The capability for stem cell potency, in combination with the relative ease to prepare bone marrow stem cell injectates, is an invaluable property for regenerative medicine cell-based therapies in general and more specifically to treat, e.g. musculoskeletal disorders (MSK-D), chronic wounds, and critical limb ischemia.

2.1 Non-embryotic autologous adult stem cells

Non-ESCs are undifferentiated, and their proliferation potential compared to embryogenic stem cells is limited, as they have lost their pluripotent capability, placing them lower in the stem cell hierarchy. Nonetheless, it has been suggested that non-ESCs maintain their multipotent differentiation potential. Since they are categorized as allogenic products, they are commercially prepared from several allogenic sources, like amniotic fluid, umbilical cord, and Wharton's jelly [3]. In this chapter we will only deliberate on non-embryotic, autologous adult bone marrow aspirate (BMA)-derived progenitor/stem cells and other bone marrow (BM) stromal cells, prepared at POC with dedicated and approved centrifuges for BM concentration.

2.2 Bone marrow-derived stromal cells

Friedenstein and colleagues reported first on the isolation of bone marrow-derived stem cells from BM stroma and incubated it in plastic culture dishes and identified mesenchymal stem cells as colony-forming unit fibroblasts (CFU-Fs) [4]. The BM stroma is made up of a network of fibroblast-like cells and includes a subpopulation of multipotent cells which are able to generate the mesenchyme, known as the mass of tissue, that develops mainly from the mesoderm of the embryo subpopulation. The cells are referred to as mesenchymal stem cells (MSCs) [5]. The *Friedenstein* culture method revealed that MSCs are capable of differentiating into several connective tissue cell types [6], described first by Pittenger and associates [7].

3. Bone marrow anatomical structure

The bone is an organ composed of cortical and trabecular bone, cartilage, and hematopoietic and connective tissues. The bone tissue has an essential role in the structure and protection of the human body. Spongy, or trabecular bone, is composed of a lattice of fine bone plates filled with hematopoietic marrow, fat-containing marrow, and arterial-venous sinusoidal blood vessels. Furthermore, it consists of bone cells at different developmental stages (including pre-osteoblasts, osteoblasts, and osteocytes), collagen fibrils, and calcium and phosphate deposits [8]. Arterial vessels enter the marrow through foramina nutricia and then divide into several arterioles. Small arterioles and capillaries from these vessels span throughout the bone marrow and supply sinusoids, which are interconnected by inter-sinusoidal capillaries [9]. The BM tissue is soft, similar to the peripheral blood, flexible connective tissue comprising the center and the epiphysis of bones, referred to as the BM cavity. In this place a variety of new blood cells are produced and ultimately released to the peripheral circulation.

3.1 Red and yellow bone marrow

We recognize two categories of bone marrow tissue: the red and yellow marrow. Depending on age, teh red marrow is replaced by the yellow marrow. In adults, the red bone marrow is a rich source of bone marrow-derived cells and present in most skeletal system bones of the iliac crest, tibia, spine vertebrae, humerus, calcaneus, ribs, and near point of attachment of long bones of legs and arms. In this well-shielded environment, an estimate of 500 billion cells per day can be produced, in particular erythrocytes, granulocytes, and platelets [10]. Regenerative medicine applications have a focus on the use of the red bone marrow as it contains myeloid and lymphoid stem cells and MSCs. In contrast the yellow marrow consists primarily of fat cells with poor vascularity and is deprived of the multipotential MSCs [11].

3.2 Bone marrow-specific regions

The BM cavity in the trabecular bone is subdivided into four regions: endosteal, sub-endosteal, central, and perisinusoidal regions [12]. In **Figure 1**, the four regions, according to the model of Lambertsen and Weis, have been adopted and modified [13]. In general, the bone marrow consists of a hematopoietic component (parenchyma) and a vascular component (stroma). The parenchyma includes hematopoietic progenitor and hematopoietic stem cells (HSCs), which are localized close to the endosteum and around the blood vessels. BM stroma cells, including endothelial cells, are recognized as multipotential non-hematopoietic progenitor cells, capable of differentiating into various tissues of mesenchymal origin, including osteoblasts, chondrocytes, tenocytes, endothelial cells, myocytes, fibroblasts, nerves, and adipocytes, as verified in in vitro and partially in in vivo research [14, 15]. The bone marrow's microvasculature includes single layers of endothelium arising in sinusoids, where they also contribute in rolling extravasations of leukocytic cells into and out of the BM tissue structures. The function of the vasculature and BM-derived endothelial cells is that they provide a barrier between the BM compartment as a functional and spatial entity from the extra-lymphoid BM section and the peripheral circulation, as described by Kopp et al. [9]. The endothelial cells likewise contribute

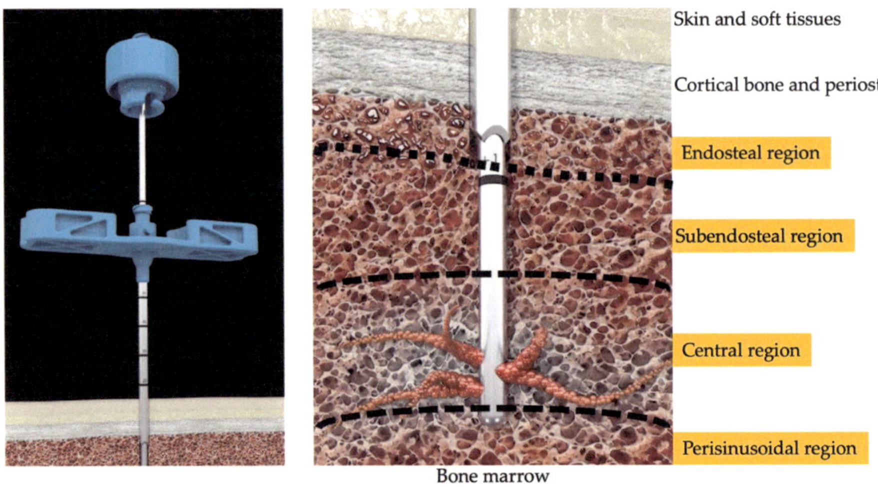

Figure 1.
Bone marrow subdivisions. On the left side, the Aspire introducer (Aspire Bone Marrow Harvesting System™, EmCyte Corporation, Fort Myers, FL, USA) has passed the cortical bone entering the marrow cavity. The harvesting cannula is inserted through the introducer in the marrow cavity. On the right side, a representation of the subdivisions in the bone marrow cavity subdivisions is indicated, showing the endosteal, sub-endosteal, central, and perisinusoidal regions. The endosteal and sub-endosteal regions compose the endosteal niche, harboring the proliferative and quiescent HSC-MSC niches. The marrow tissue is extracted via the side holes of the harvesting cannula (adapted and modified from Lambertsen and Weis [13]).

to tissue regeneration, as endothelial precursor cells are essential in improving vascularization of damaged and degenerative tissue cells by the secretion of pro-angiopoietic factors of invading cells [16].

3.3 Bone marrow niches

A *niche* is defined by anatomy and function. Stem cell niches are defined as specific cellular and molecular microenvironments regulating stem cell and progenitor functions. A niche consists of signaling molecules, intercellular contact, and the interaction between stem cells and their neighboring extracellular matrix (ECM). This three-dimensional microenvironment is thought to control genes and properties that define "stemness," including the control and balance between quiescence, self-renewal, proliferation, and differentiation of diverse cell types. Additionally, the microenvironment provides stem cell autonomous signaling mechanisms [17, 18], and it engages in specific cascades to a stress response [19]. Acquired and prepared BM stem cells from one of the niches and subsequently injected into a totally different microenvironment can potentially differentiate into cell types of this new environment [20]. Zhao et al. used a rat stroke model in which BM-MSCs were transplanted into neural tissues. They demonstrated that MSCs originating from the BM-MSC niche differentiated into neuronal cells after transplantation into the neural microenvironment [21]. Their observation revealed the plasticity potential of BM-MSCs, as well as the possible influence of the recipient niche, as BM-MSCs were capable of dedifferentiation into cells from other cell lineages. Their finding has potentially significant clinical implications for regenerative medicine applications overall. Since autologously prepared MSCs originate from their specific and original BM niche but are used in other cellular tissue types to treat various pathologies, they can be successfully engaged in tissue repair and regeneration through regenerative medicine application techniques. This is a distinctly different approach in the physiological release of newly formed BM cells, because they are retained in the BM cavity until they mature and thereafter released in the vascular peripheral circulation [15].

3.3.1 Hematopoietic and mesenchymal niche

HSC niches are present in various (prenatal) tissues, like the aorta-gonad-mesonephros region and the yolk sac, followed by the placenta, fetal liver, spleen, and bone marrow. Postnatally, the bone marrow is the primary site of HSC presence [22]. The model of the HSC niche was first described by Schofield in 1978 [23], later confirmed by others, to describe the physiologically limited microenvironment in which HSCs, MSCs, and their progenitors reside in the bone cavity where they are enfolded by BM stromal cells [24], covered by the bony structure of the BM cavity. The stem cell niches in bone have been extensively described by Yin and Li, providing insights into the actions of osteoblastic and vascular niches, revealing central roles for numerous signaling and adhesion molecules [25]. A significant portion of these hematopoietic cells is found next to the endosteal bone surface, designating a clear role for osteoblasts in the regulation of HSCs and thus hematopoiesis [26]. Based on flow cytometry research by Kiel et al., HSCs are more likely than other hematopoietic cells to be immediately adjacent to a sinusoid, in the trabecular region of the BM [27]. This location suggests that HSCs and their niche may be directly, or indirectly, regulated by factors present near the bone planes. The HSC niche is comprised of many different niche constituents including osteoclasts, endothelial cells, fibroblasts, adipocytes, and the HSC progenitor cells [28].

3.3.2 Perivascular niche

The BM is highly vascularized, with large central arteries branching into progressively smaller microvessels like arterioles and transitioning into venous sinusoids near the bone (endosteal) surface. Therefore, it has been suggested that HSCs are maintained in a perivascular niche by endothelial or perivascular cells, as they are frequently located adjacent to the blood vessels [29]. These occurrences resulted in the expression of various perivascular mesenchymal cell makers CD146, stromal cell-derived factor-1 (SDF-1) also referred to as CXCL12, and Nestin-GFP, defining the heterogenous BM stroma cell composition [9], including the MSCs that surround the blood vessels [30]. The more perivascular nature of MSC niches was validated by Shi and Gronthos, demonstrating the expression of α-smooth muscle actin (αSMA) at perivascular sites, with the immunohistochemical localization of specific CD marker cells [31]. Mores studies confirmed the presence of MSCs in BM, expressing a Nestin-GFP transgene, localized and attached around the BM blood vessels and part of the perivascular HSC niche [32]. Kunisaki et al. indicated that most HSCs do not only have a perivascular presence, but they are preferentially located in the BM endosteal regions. The endosteal regions contain a complex network of stromal cells as well that have been implicated in HSC maintenance, including arteriolar and venous endothelial cells, pericytes, and chemokine (C-X-C) ligand 12 (CXCL12) reticular cells. Their study also suggested that quiescent HSCs localize preferentially to small arterioles near the endosteum, suggesting that distinct niches may exist for both quiescent and proliferating HSCs [33]. From all these findings, it can be concluded that pericytes are in fact MSCs, because they can differentiate in osteoblasts, chondrocytes, and adipocytes [34].

3.3.3 Megakaryocyte niche

Megakaryocytes (MK) are the precursor cells of blood platelets. BM hematopoietic cells are responsible for platelet production. MK may regulate HSCs indirectly as they are closely associated with BM sinusoidal endothelium, extending cytoplasmic protrusions into the sinusoids to produce platelets. A direct regulation of HSC by MK through signaling of transforming growth factor beta 1 was established, with activation of quiescent HSCs and increased proliferation rate. In the event of a sudden response to systemic stress signaling, fibroblast growth factor-1 as part of the MK growth factor pool will start signaling HSCs and will overshadow the TGF-b1 signaling in order to stimulate high volumes of HSC expansion [35].

3.4 Extracellular matrix

The role and function of the extracellular matrix (ECM) can be defined as key structural-functional components of cell niches, including soluble factors, cell-cell contacts, and cell-matrix adhesions present in these microenvironments. ECM components include fibrillar proteins, with, among others, collagen fibers, fibronectin, and other filamentous network components. The ECM's mechanical stability is provided by collagen [36]. Other significant ECM components supporting the BM niches are glycosaminoglycans and mainly hyaluronic acid via its receptor CD44. The surface marker is also expressed by MSCs and HSCs [37]. Intracellular signaling in the ECM occurs through cytokine and growth factor membrane receptors, similar to the MSC niche. These cytokines and receptor activities contribute to cross talk between ECM components and MSC niches, provoking cell differentiation. For instance, Djouad et al. demonstrated that the induction of MSC differentiation towards chondrocytes in articular cartilage was induced and/or influenced by molecules from both the MSC niche and the ECM components of this microenvironment, leading to chondrogenic differentiation of MSCs [38]. Other studies suggested that ECM deposited by microvascular endothelial cells enhances MSC endotheliogenesis [39]. In general, no specific ECM components are identified that maintain MSCs in their immature state, as a niche matrix would do. However, it has become clear that the ECM can regulate MSC differentiation on a solitary basis, indicating potential applications for regenerative medicine applications and tissue engineering.

4. Bone marrow aspiration procedures

Exploiting BM preparations at POC seeks to overcome the limitations of ex vivo MSC culturing. Clinicians utilizing regenerative medicine applications have a growing interest in using the concentrated bone marrow products, since it is well acknowledged that BM is a plentiful source of MSCs, progenitors, and other cells residing in the trabecular part of flat and long bones, acquired via appropriately performed BMA procedures [40, 41]. The regenerative medicine market is rapidly growing, with many procedures performed in musculoskeletal, orthopedic, and spinal disorders, wound care management including critical limb ischemia, and tissue engineering [42–45]. Several groups have mentioned some considerations when performing BM harvesting procedures, addressing a variety of factors that have an impact on patient comfort and the quality of the harvested BM. Emphasis was given to procedural safety issues when using harvesting needle systems, level of experience of the operator, the choice for concentration technology and centrifugation devices, and pain management [46]. Autologous regenerative medicine BM-MSC applications may range from a harvesting a low volume of BM and direct, unprocessed, tissue injection to the use of centrifugation protocols to concentrate and filter the BMA prior to injecting it in patients [47].

4.1 Bone marrow harvesting needle systems

Various bone marrow needle harvesting systems are available on the market, each with their own proprietary design characteristics and thus marrow aspiration dynamics when transferring marrow cavity cells through a needle system into collection syringes. In **Figure 2**, three different needle systems are shown. Potentially, different needle design features might affect the quality and viability of the harvested BM tissue, as well as the cellular yields. Therefore, BM needle system features and harvesting dynamics are important considerations when considering BMA procedures. Physicians have been using a variety of harvesting needles during the last decades, including the traditional Jamshidi™ harvesting needle (Ranfac Corporation, Avon, MA, USA). Based on design differences, not every BMA is born equal, and cellular yields, composition, and viability might vary among harvesting devices. For interpretation purposes, some of the cellular difference between two newly developed BMA needle harvesting systems, the Aspire Bone Marrow Harvesting System™ and the Marrow Cellution Bone Marrow Aspiration Device™ (EmCyte Corporation, Fort Myers, FL, USA, and Ranfac Corporation, Avon, MA, USA, respectively) is shown. A significant difference between the two harvesting

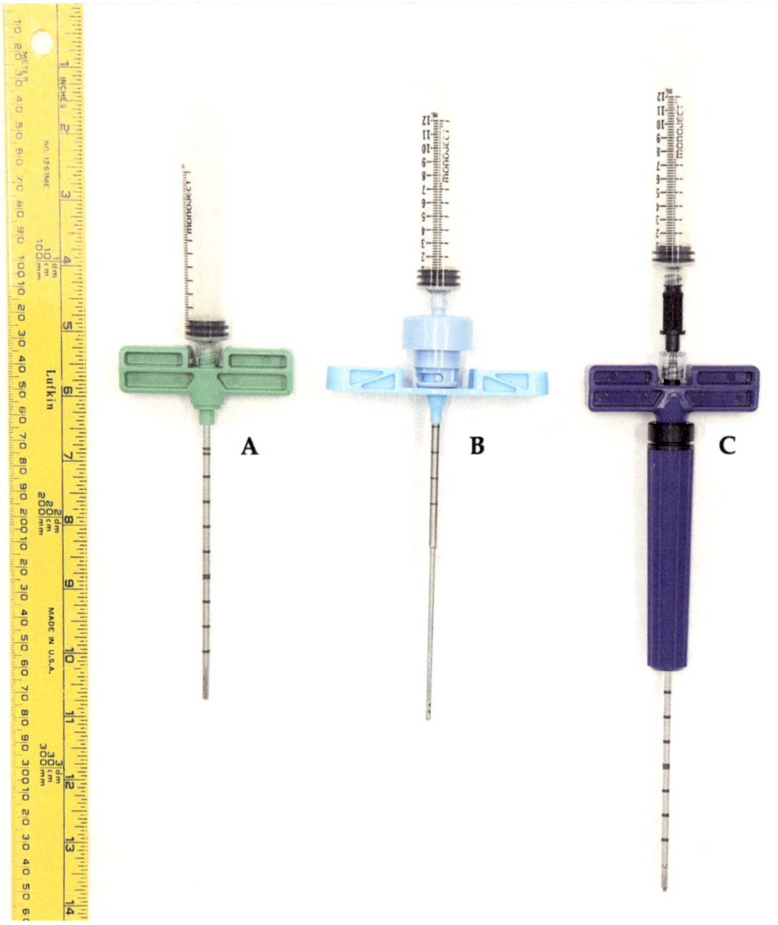

Figure 2.
Bone marrow aspiration devices. (A) Jamshidi™ device (Ranfac Corporation, Avon, MA, USA), with a sharp and open distal tip, allows for more peripheral blood aspiration. (B) Aspire Bone Marrow Harvesting System™ (EmCyte Corporation, Fort Myers, FL, USA) consists of a separate trocar introducer and aspiration needle with a completely closed and blunt tip. The side holes of the aspiration needle are designed to minimize cellular trauma and hemolysis during aspiration. (C) Marrow Cellution Bone Marrow Aspiration Device™ (Ranfac Corporation, Avon, MA, USA) is used as an aspiration device only, to aspirate 10 ml of bone marrow, followed by unfiltered injection.

systems is that the Marrow Cellution device is developed and used by physicians for BMA aspiration with direct injection only, without filtration or processing prior to patient injection [47]. Therefore, these specimens mimic the marrow cavity cellular content and their specific cell concentrations. This includes a red blood cell (RBC) content and hematocrit which is similar to the peripheral blood values. Conditional negative forces occur with the syringe pull during marrow aspiration; this particular BMA injectate can have high plasma-free hemoglobin (PFH) concentrations, which cannot be removed from the injectate. The Aspire™ harvesting system is designed to penetrate the trabecular bone, maintaining a quiescent tissue environment during deployment and collection, contributing to a reduction in tissue activation, plasma-free hemoglobin content, and clotting. The Aspire™ harvesting system is intended to provide a BMA for centrifugation processing, leading in this occasion to the creation of PurePRP SupraPhysiologic BMC® (EmCyte Corporation, Fort Myers, FL, USA). In **Table 1**, comparative laboratory data between the abovementioned needle systems in a bilateral patient harvesting model are disclosed.

Laboratory parameters	BMA-MC 10 ml	BMA-A 10 ml	BMC 11 ml
TNC × 10^6/mL	25.8	31.8	73.7
Platelets × 10^6/mL	117	117	576
CD34+ (HSCs) × 10^5/mL	1.42	1.12	2.51
CFU-F (MSCs) × 10^3/mL	446	1.13	837
Hematocrit %	36.2	36.2	9.8
RBCs × 10^9/mL	4.02	4.08	1.44
PFH mg/dl	913	721	299
Hemolysis %	4.6	3.2	1.6
Cell viability %	94.4	94.4	96.8

BMA-MC, bone marrow aspirate Marrow Cellution System; BMA-A, bone marrow aspirate Aspire System; BMC, bone marrow concentrate; TNC, total nucleated cells; CD34+, hematopoietic stem cell marker/expression in bone marrow; CFU-F, colony-forming unit fibroblast: assay for bone marrow mesenchymal stem cell analysis, MSCs, mesenchymal stem cells. (BMA-MC, Marrow Cellution Device™—Ranfac Corporation, Avon, MA, USA; BMA-A, Aspire Bone Marrow Harvesting System™—EmCyte Corporation, Fort Myers, FL, USA).

Table 1.
Comparative quantification between two different bone marrow aspiration systems and bone marrow concentrate, in a bilateral patient model.

4.2 Large vs. small BMA collection syringes

In theory, a larger-volume BMA collection syringe should produce a stronger negative pressure and therefore harvest more MSCs. However, Hernigou et al. found that the aspiration of only 10–20% of the full syringe volume resulted in a higher MSC concentration in both 10 and 50 ml syringes, indicating that high-quality harvesting of MSCs requires a significant negative pressure in the marrow cavity to liberate MSCs. They also concluded that the collection of MSCs decreased as the syringe was filled, at a lower negative pressure [40]. Therefore, smaller syringes and thus smaller aspiration volumes result in higher MSC concentrations than with larger aspiration volumes [48]. This translates to the physical equation, "Negative Pressure = Pull Force/Plunger Surface Area," resulting in the fact that with the same pull force and a smaller diameter syringe plunger, a higher negative pressure is created [49]. Lately, the authors use 10 ml syringes, employing a fast and intermittent pull technique to collect small volumes from different intra-trabecular sites (**Figure 3**). This is in accordance with a trend towards small-volume HPD aspiration techniques [50]. Another advantage for using 10 ml syringes is that anticoagulation protocols can be better managed. Smaller syringes fill considerably quicker than larger syringes, and smaller syringes can be adequately agitated with the anticoagulant to avoid clotting.

4.3 Image-guided aspiration

In order to perform BM-MSC procedures, a certain volume and quality of marrow tissue are required in order to prepare a bone marrow concentrate (BMC). The aspiration volume is contingent on the processing volume of the BMC concentration system that is being used. It is imperative to locate precisely the donor site, as MSCs are located in the marrow cavity subcortical area and around the blood vessels [19]. The precise delivery of local anesthetics and safe trocar placement are accomplished by using image guidance during aspiration procedure. In the following section, we focus on the posterior super iliac spine (PSIS) sites, as it is the most frequently reported anatomical site for BMA.

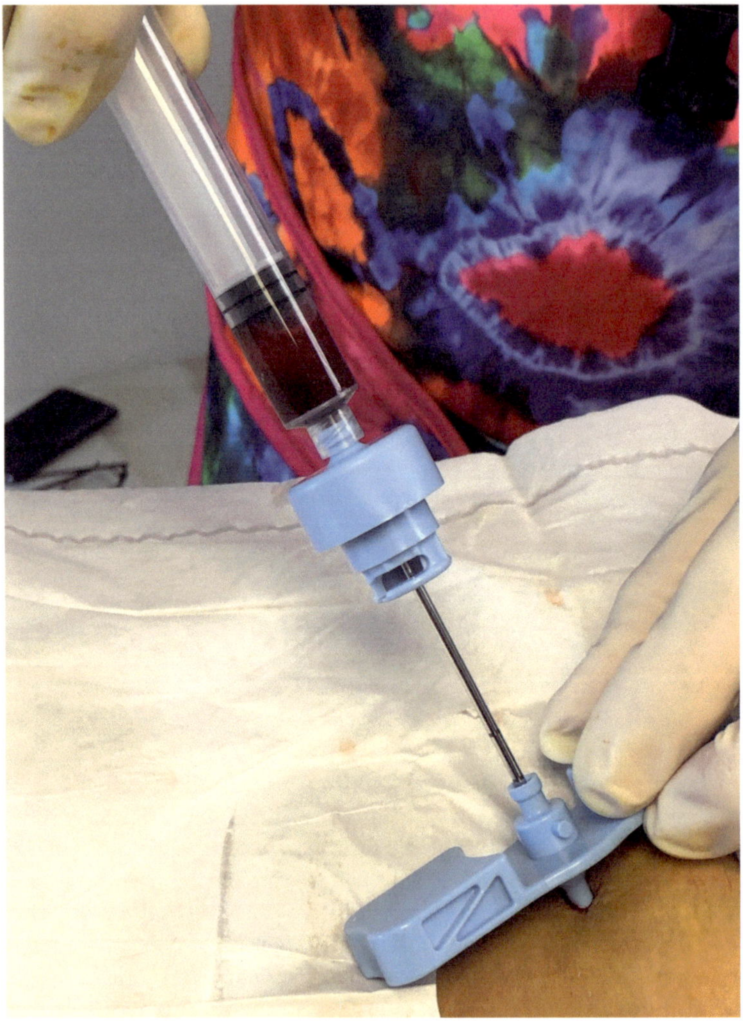

Figure 3.
Bone marrow aspiration. After the aspiration needle has been advanced in the marrow cavity, the marrow is extracted using a firm, but a gentle, aspiration pressure is applied to the 10 ml syringe. The aspiration needle is easily rotated to collect marrow from a fresh area.

4.3.1 Ultrasound imaging

When the PSIS is targeted, patients are positioned in the prone position, while avoiding lumbar lordosis. Sonographic assessment using a portable ultrasound system with a 5–2 MHz low-frequency curvilinear transducer is positioned in a transverse plane over the hyperechoic bilateral sacral cornua, with the patient lying prone and the monitor screen in the line of sight of the operator. The probe is then translated contralaterally from the physician, keeping the hyperechoic sacrum visualized. Next, the probe is translated proximally, with the hyperechoic ilium coming into view, while maintaining the hyperechoic sacrum, until the most superficial depth of the ilium is reached, known as the PSIS, contralateral to the examiner [51]. After identification of the PSIS, the most superficial depth is confirmed in both transverse and longitudinal orientation (**Figure 4**). With the probe in the transverse plane at the PSIS, the slope of the iliac wing is noted for correct angulation of the BM trocar, and the most superficial depth of the PSIS is brought under the most medial aspect of the ultrasound probe. Using a sterile marker, a mark and

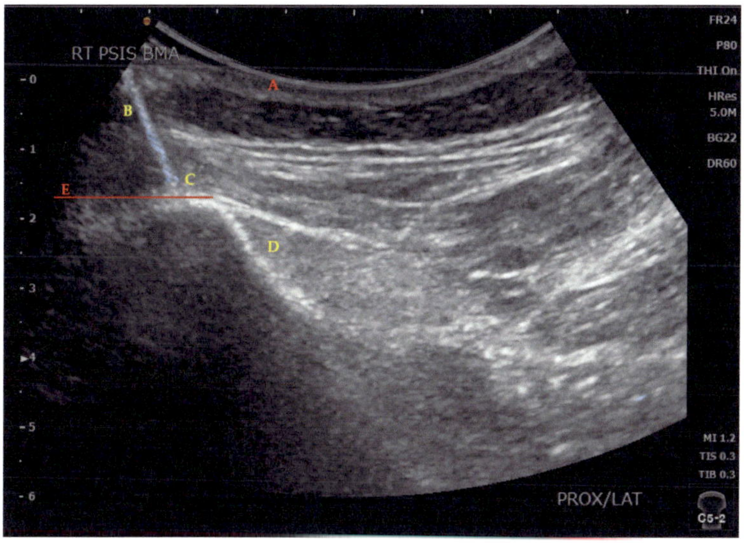

Figure 4.
Ultrasound imaging of the PSIS. With the probe in the transverse plane, the PSIS is confirmed, and the slope (D) of the iliac wing is noted for correct angulation of the BM trocar (B), and the most superficial depth (C) of the PSIS is brought under the most medial aspect of the ultrasound probe. Note: (A) indicates the skin surface, and (E) marks the depth of the PSIS below the skin, in this patient approximately 1.6 cm (courtesy of J. Rothenberg).

directional line is made in both parallel and perpendicular orientations to form an intersection at the most superficial depth of the PSIS. This mark is maintained on the patient during skin preparation prior to the introduction off the BM trocar, and a superficial wheal of local anesthetic is placed at the point of planned trocar skin entry. Following the local antiseptic measures, sterile ultrasound gel is applied at the marked area, and a sterile probe cover is applied to the 5–2 MHz curvilinear array transducer. Typically, a mixture of local anesthetics is injected around the PSIS cortex and periosteal sleeve, under continued sonographic guidance, making sure to "walk off" the PSIS in four directions (superiorly, medially, laterally, and inferiorly), confirmed by sonographic guidance. The trocar is then introduced, using either a manual force that is perpendicular and slightly lateral to the patient, at 9–12 counterclockwise-clockwise rotations, or a mallet. The next steps of the procedure are subject to the implementation of the instructions for use provided by the manufacturer of the aspiration harvesting system.

4.3.2 Fluoroscopic imaging

After proper patient positioning, the fluoroscopic equipment is installed to optimize the positioning for fluoroscopic imaging, using ipsilateral or contralateral oblique beam angulations for viewing the targeted PSIS site. The *perpendicular fluoroscopic approach* requires a beam angle around 15° ipsilateral to the PSIS entering laterally with angulation towards the sacroiliac joint. This angle will view the lateral ilium outer wall, and a needle is directed anteromedially. Fluoroscopic images support in positioning the tip of the trocar above the target area for entering the PSIS. The *parallel fluoroscopic approach* results in viewing down the PSIS table, at a 25° contralateral oblique beam position. This results in a classic view of the "teardrop" (**Figure 5**). Imaging can confirm the entry point into the PSIS table and visualize the angle through the cortex, allowing for safe trocar advancement in the BM cavity, at the tick part of the ilium bone [52]. Using proper fluoroscopic

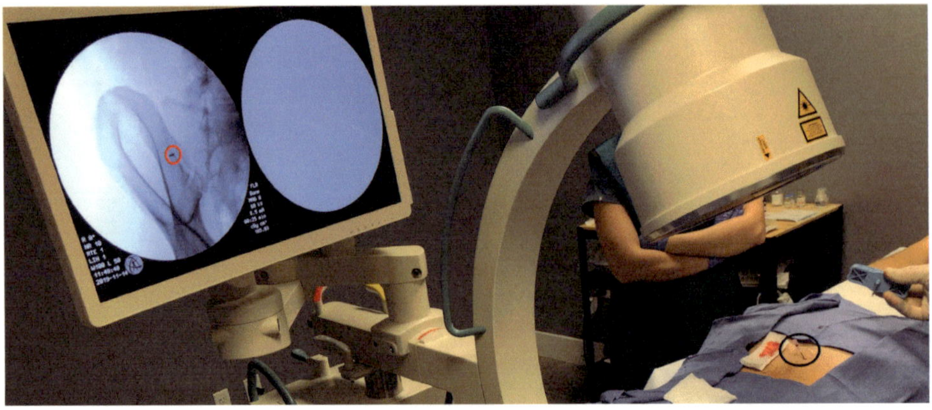

Figure 5.
Fluoroscopy imaging of the PSIS. General prone position of the patient on a fluoroscopic table for BMA. The parallel fluoroscopic approach *results in viewing down the PSIS table, at a 25° contralateral oblique beam position. This results in a classic view of the "teardrop," referring to the outline of the medial and lateral borders, as shown in the monitor. The tip of a needle (black circle), in the numbed skin, is marking the entry site of the bone marrow trocar to be placed in the marrow cavity, while the physician is on the ipsilateral side of the fluoroscope, viewing the correct position on the monitor (red circle) (courtesy of G. Flanagan II).*

techniques, the parallel approach technique allows for a safe deeper marrow penetration. However, at all times, regardless of the approach, avoid increased manipulation and tissue trauma using the sharp trocar, as this will increase the risk for neurovascular injury, bleeding, tearing of lateral gluteal muscle origins, and post-procedural pain.

4.4 Bone marrow aspiration anatomical sites

As MSCs represent a small population of BM cells [7], it is of critical importance to choose a BMA site that will yield the most MSCs. BM is relatively easy to harvest, largely available, and dispensable. Obviously, it is important that the BMA procedure is performed impeccably to obtain an optimal quality of viable BM tissue [5, 53]. In humans, the most common anatomical location to obtain BM is the iliac crest, but other BMA sites have been utilized (**Table 2**). Recently, McDaniel and co-workers, using a porcine model, reported that all studied anatomical bone marrow harvesting locations contained MSCs but the iliac crest was the most abundant

Anterior superior iliac spine (ASIS)
Posterior superior iliac spine (PSIS)
Proximal tibia
Distal tibia
Distal femur
Proximal humerus
Vertebral body
Calcaneus
Sternum

Table 2.
Bone marrow aspiration sites in humans.

source of MSCs [10]. These findings were confirmed in a clinical study, where MSCs were found in BM acquired from the metaphysis of the distal femur, the proximal tibia, and iliac crest. A similar MSC immunophenotype and differentiation potential (into the bone, fat, and cartilage) were seen in BMA from all sites. However, in their study the concentration of MSCs in the iliac crest was significantly higher than in samples from the distal femur and proximal tibia. More specifically, the literature indicates high yields of BM-MSCs acquired from the posterior superior iliac spine (PSIS) [50, 54]. Noteworthy, the group of Narbona-Carceles commented on the relative easiness and safety of lower extremity aspiration techniques [55].

5. Major type of cells in bone marrow

The literature pronounces BMAs as a heterogenous mix of cells, referring in most instances to MSCs, HSCs, and mononuclear cells. Platelets, megakaryocytes, and RBCs are seldomly mentioned, let be subject to BM research [24].

5.1 Hematopoietic stem cells

The major function of the bone marrow is to generate blood cells. In particular in adults, marrow-derived HSCs are the principle cells of origin of all mature hematopoietic cell phenotypes. HSCs are adult stem cells with extensive self-renewal capabilities and are able to differentiate into specialized blood cells with key roles in some biological activities: control homeostasis balance, immune functions, and response to microorganisms and inflammation. Most HSCs are in a quiescent state within the BM niches. They respond to the signals after the balance of blood cells, or HSC pool, is disturbed from either intrinsic or extrinsic stimuli and signaling processes [56].

5.1.1 Hematopoiesis

Hematopoiesis—the process by which mature blood cells are formed—has been studied intensely for over a century. The vast majority of hematopoiesis occurs in the bone marrow where it must balance enormous production needs. More than 500 billion blood cells are produced every day, with precise regulation of the number of each blood cell type released in the circulation [57]. Hematopoiesis is considered as a pyramidal/hierarchical process with cells of greatest maturation potential or primitiveness sitting at the top of the hierarchy and cells that have undergone terminal differentiation at the bottom. Terminally differentiated blood cells are classified into one of the two major lineages: those derived from myeloid lineages and from lymphoid progenitors. Myeloid cells include erythrocytes, platelets, and cells responsible for cellular immunity, such as macrophages and granulocytes (**Figure 6**). Cells derived from lymphoid progenitors are major participants in coordinating humeral and cellular immunity. Experimental data suggested that HSCs differentiate into hematopoietic progenitor cells that are capable of exponential proliferation as well as continuing the process of differentiation. Alternatively, HSCs are capable of self-replicating activities, which may give rise to one or two identical daughter cells. As a result, HSC activity must be tightly regulated to meet physiologic demands but also to protect HSCs from oncogenic, physical, and chemical damage to occur. The site or physical location that regulates self-renewal, proliferation, and differentiation of HSCs has been discussed in the HSC niche paragraph.

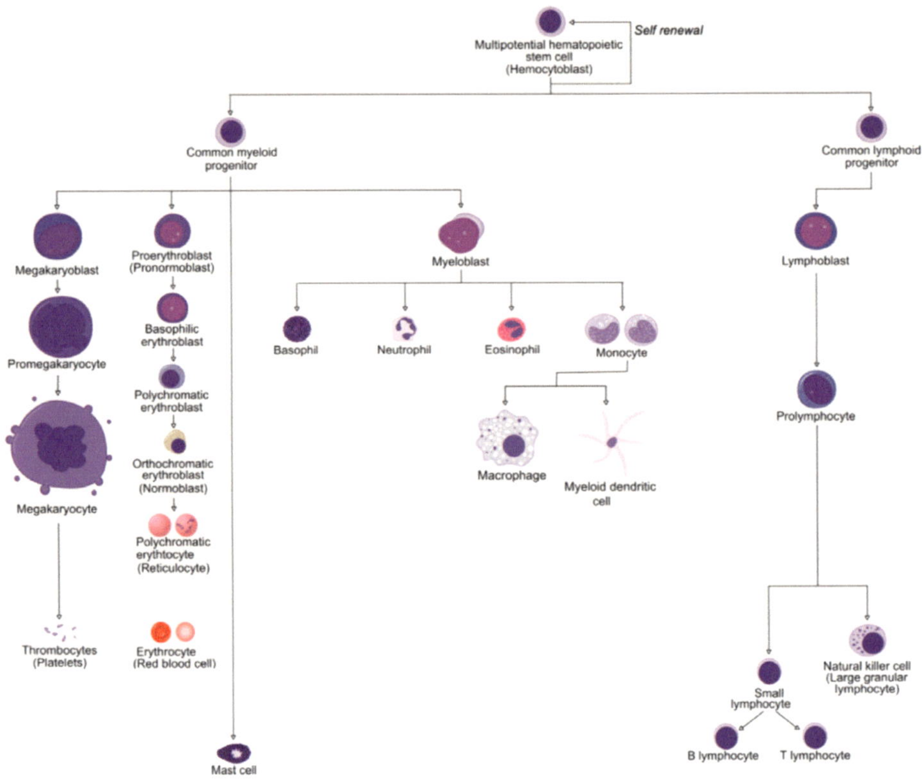

Figure 6.
Hematopoietic stem cell hierarchy. Self-renewing HSCs give rise to common myeloid progenitors and common lymphoid progenitors, producing different types of progenitor cells and ultimately fully differentiated cells. The myeloid progenitors produce granulocyte-macrophage progenitors giving rise to differentiated leukocytic cells and mast cells. The megakaryocyte/erythrocyte progenitors give rise to megakaryocytes, platelets, and erythrocytes. The lymphoid progenitors differentiate ultimately in lymphocytic cell variances.

5.1.2 HSC and angiogenesis

Emerging evidence suggests that BM-derived endothelial cells and HSCs, including their progenitor cells, contribute to tissue vascularization. HSCs deliver specific angiogenetic factors, facilitating the incorporation of endothelial progenitor cells into newly sprouting vessels. Several clinical studies have shown that BM-derived cells contribute to neo-angiogenesis during wound healing [44], critical limb ischemia [45], and postmyocardial infarction [58]. This should contribute to the clinical discussion of the value of BM-derived HSC and vascular progenitor as they are able to contribute to tissue restoration by accelerating tissue vascularization and regeneration [15, 59].

5.2 Mesenchymal stem cells

In recent decades, physicians performing regenerative medicine applications have been more interested in the potential of BM-MSCs than of HSCs. Imaginable reasons for this particular interest in MSCs might be recent published expert opinions: the *in vivo* ability of MSCs to migrate into tissues, their sturdy regenerative and reparative properties, and the MSC-mediated immunomodulatory actions.

These typical characteristics and particular mode of actions enable conceivable BM cell-based treatment options [60, 61]. In particular, MSCs do not express significant histocompatibility complexes and immune-stimulating molecules, leading to graft rejection. Likewise, a rapid development in clinical outcome reporting, with a better understanding of BM tissue molecular biology, improved bone marrow aspiration techniques and, at POC BM concentration and preparation methods, has increased the interest and demand for autologous BM stem and progenitor cell therapies.

5.2.1 MSC isolation procedure from bone marrow aspirates

An effective BM-MSC injection is reliant on the performance of the marrow aspiration procedure, minimizing cellular trauma, while maximizing cellular yields and simultaneously avoiding peripheral RBC infiltration [62]. BM aspiration procedures, and not diagnostics, are routinely performed to collect bone marrow tissue to be processed using dedicated BM-MSC concentration kits for regenerative medicine applications. Kits may include a harvesting needle system and/or BM concentration device (**Figure 7**). These at POC MSC isolation techniques are a streamlined method to concentrate marrow cells, including MSCs, HSCs, and progenitor cells. These MSC centrifugation procedures demand less time and attention than laboratory preparation and culturing methodologies which are technically demanding. Double-spin centrifugation protocols create a layered BMC buffy coat stratum, based on different centrifugal forces that accomplish density cellular separation, as a result of the specific cellular gravity of the individual marrow components, as shown in **Figure 8**. Furthermore, BMA concentration-based technologies provide an economic and clinical/patient advantage when compared to the culturing technologies.

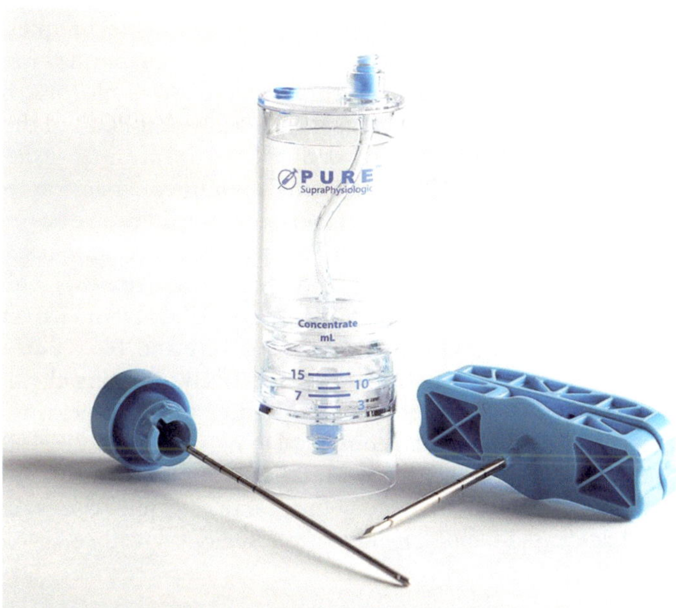

Figure 7.
Bone marrow preparation essential components. In bone marrow concentration and preparation kits, the foremost components are a bone marrow harvesting needle and a concentration device (courtesy of EmCyte Corporation, Fort Myers, FL, USA).

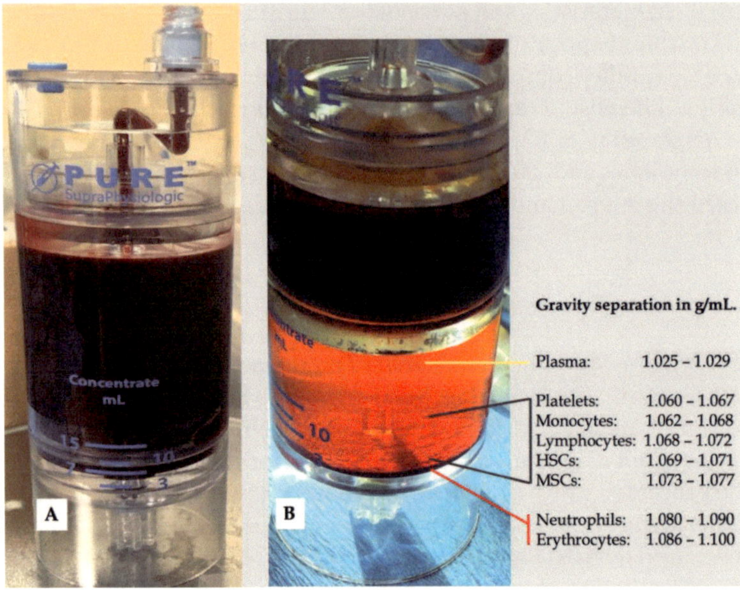

Figure 8.
Bone marrow gravity separation following centrifugation. (A) Bone marrow aspirate in concentration device before centrifugation. In (B), the bone marrow aspirate is concentrated, with a view on the buffy coat stratum (gray layer on top of the RBC layer), referenced by the two black lines. Following a two-step centrifugation protocol, the centrifugal forces achieve density marrow cell separation due to the specific gravities of the individual marrow components.

5.2.2 MSC culturing protocols

Traditionally, BM-MSCs have been separated from other BM cells following strict laboratory cell processing protocols. These cell processing techniques are lengthy procedures, as they cannot be performed at POC, as a same-day procedure. In many parts of the world, clinicians are allowed to use autologous, fresh, and non-cultured BMA and BMC products that are prepared at POC. In the USA, regenerative medicine biological procedures demand the use of the so-called 510-K FDA-approved devices. The use of MSCs following laboratory expansion techniques is facing considerable legislative barriers. Furthermore, the literature has cited potential risks associated with laboratory MSC cell processing techniques, like tumorigenicity [63], genetic instability [64], and immunogenicity [65]. Others raise concern regarding the efficacy and function of cultured MSCs by in vitro culture conditions during the cell passages for cell expansion. Karp and Teo reported on the loss of specific MSC surface receptors functions, negatively affecting chemotaxis [66]. Others have informed on impaired homing abilities and disappearing CXCR4 receptors following cell culturing, when compared to non-cultured BMA, in which high CXCR4 concentrations were measured [67]. Last but not least, laboratory MSC cell culturing methods for regenerative medicine practices require the availability of a specialized and dedicated facility, using strict regulatory protocols which will increase costs [68].

5.2.3 Characterization of bone marrow mesenchymal stem cells

In order to better understand the specifics of MSC cell concentrations, counts, and quality, it's important to understand the differences between laboratory techniques analyzing HSCs and MSCs, as they differ with regard to the specificity and relevance of the different BM cell types, possibly effecting regenerative medicine therapy outcomes.

5.2.3.1 ISCT criteria

The International Society of Cellular Therapy (ISCT) has developed criteria in order to outline human MSCs for both laboratory-based scientific investigations and for preclinical studies [69]. MSCs are defined as those cells that are able to adhere to plastic and express a number of cell surface markers while undergoing multilineage differentiation [70].

5.2.3.2 Flow cytometry and CD markers

It has been difficult to determine what type of cells is neighboring both MSCs and HSCs and contributes to the regulation of the functional continuation of stem cell, as immunostaining methods are complex procedures to perform. Flow cytometry is a laboratory technique used to detect and measure characteristics of cell/particle populations by measuring their physical and chemical properties. A specific protocol for the identification of dissimilar cell surface molecules is called cluster of differentiation (CD) where monoclonal antibodies (markers) are used to establish positive and negative staining for certain cell types. Specifically for MSC and HSC, explicit CD markers are established to validate BM cellular content, as it is widely accepted that MSC cultures are a heterogenous source of cells with varying self-renewal and differentiation properties [71]. This indicates that there is no single unique indicator for identification. Hence, a panel of both positive and negative protein markers is used to identify the cell surface markers that are expressed by MSC populations, like CD29, VD44, CD51, CD73, CD90, CD105, CD166, and Stro1. While they must be negative for hematopoietic stem cell markers like CD14, CD34, and CD45 [72], some of these markers are included in the minimum ISCT criteria.

5.2.3.3 Colony-forming unit fibroblast assay

In the initial BM monolayer, several hematopoietic oriented cells (macrophages, endothelial cells, and lymphocytes) adhere to plastic [7]. Nevertheless, in culturing conditions only fibroblast-like spindle-shaped cells proliferate and form ultimately CFU-F colonies. These cells are representative of the more highly proliferative cells in MSCs [73]. The CFU-F assay is a different method used to determine the MSC presence in a vial of BM tissue. Unlike a complete blood count test, which is a quantitative blood cell analysis, the CFU-F assay is a laboratory assay in particular for stem and progenitor cell determination (**Figure 9**) [74]. The CFU-F assay is a qualitative indicator of the proliferative and differentiation capability of individual MSC cells within a BMA or BMC sample. The cells are seeded and cultured in a growth medium where they have to adhere to plastic, at 37°C. After 14 days the cultures are evaluated, and CFU-Fs are counted, whereby a minimum of 50 cells per CFU need to be defined.

5.3 MSC capacities

MSCs are multipotent stem cells which can be obtained from various adult tissues, like the BM stroma, adipose tissue, synovium, periosteum, and trabecular bone. Typical features are their ability for self-renewal, defined as sustaining

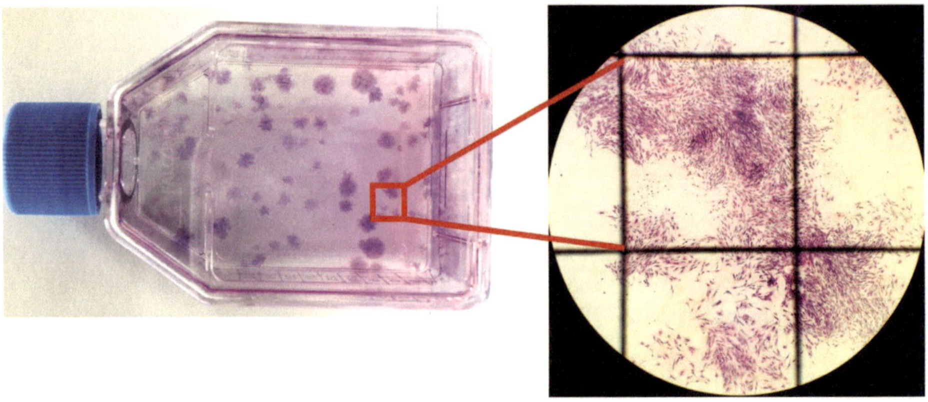

Figure 9.
MSC culturing. A picture of a flask cultured with stained human MSCs. The zoomed-in area is a light micrograph showing the morphology of a MSC colony in a patient treated with BMC. After culturing for 14 days, the MSC count in this example was 1065/mL (picture courtesy of BioSciences Research Associates, Cambridge, MA, USA).

biological pathways and mechanisms to preserve the undifferentiated stem state, and the regulation of lineage-specific differentiation [39]. Although the number of MSCs represents only a small fraction of non-hematopoietic, multipotent cells of the bone marrow (0.001–0.01%), understanding these unique cells has taken great strides forward. Generally, MSCs have developed a great attractiveness for regenerative medicine autologous therapeutic applications and tissue engineering opportunities, because of their multipotentiality and relative ease of isolation from numerous tissues, like BM [75]. MSCs can be also identified as specialized populations of mural cells or pericytes, sharing a niche with HSCs. Under appropriate conditions and an optimal microenvironment, MSCs can differentiate into various mesodermal lineages like osteoblasts, chondrocytes, endothelial cells, adipose tissue, and smooth muscle cells (**Figure 10**) [76]. These MSC proficiencies have led to the use of MSC as a potential strategy for treating various diseases, since they encourage biological processes, for example angiogenesis, cell proliferation, and cell differentiation [77]. Furthermore, they synthesize cytokines and trophic mediators which participate in tissue repair processes, immune modulation, and the regulation of inflammatory processes [78]. Caplan also suggested that the modulation of inflammation is instigated by the suppression of inflammatory T-cell proliferation and inhibition of monocyte and myeloid cell maturation [79]. Based on the above characteristics, it can be assumed that MSCs are capable to institute a regenerative microenvironment at the site of release and improve the various cell recruitment, cell-signaling, and differentiation of endogenous stem cells, with the potential to instigate tissue repair in a variety of disease states.

5.4 MSC immunomodulatory effects

In parallel with their major role as undifferentiated cell reserves, MSCs have immunomodulatory functions which are exerted by direct cell-to-cell contact, secretion of cytokines, and/or by a combination of both mechanisms. MSCs have been shown to exert profound anti-inflammatory and immunomodulatory effects on almost all the cells of the innate and adaptive immune systems via a variety of mechanisms, notably cytokine and chemokine secretion [80]. The immunosuppressive capabilities of MSCs are only exploited when they are exposed to sufficiently high concentrations of pro-inflammatory cytokines, like interferon-gamma (IFN-γ), tissue necrosis factor α, (TNF- α), and interleukins α or ß (IL-1α, IL ß).

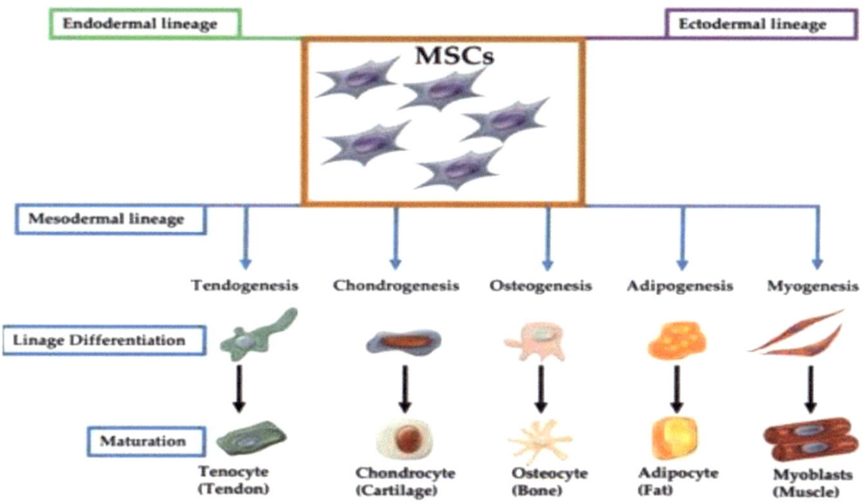

Figure 10.
MSC differentiation potential. MSC differentiation potential into endodermal, ectodermal, and mesodermal lineages. The mesodermal lineage differentiation has been recognized as the most attractive differentiation lineages for regenerative medicine applications, executed at point of care, as these produce osteoblasts, chondrocytes, tenocytes, adipose tissues, and smooth muscle cells.

In order for MSCs to become "immunosuppressants," they need to be triggered by these inflammatory cytokines, and the inflammatory environment is then a crucial factor for MSCs to exert their immunomodulatory effects. These are wielded by blocking apoptosis of native and activated neutrophils, aside from decreasing neutrophils from binding to vascular endothelial cells and the mobilization of neutrophils to the area of damage [81]. Furthermore, MSCs constrain the complement-mediated effects of peripheral blood mononuclear cell proliferation [82], and they limit mast cell degranulation and the secretion of pro-inflammatory cytokines, while at the same time MSCs migrate towards CXCL12 and other chemotactic factors [83]. In **Figure 11** the MSC cell-dependent trophic support mechanisms are shown. Data from Jiang and others suggested that MSCs can block the differentiation of CD34+ cells from BM or blood monocytes into mature dendritic cells by direct contact as well as by secreted paracrine factors [84]. Under their influence, M1 (pro-inflammatory) macrophages are transformed into M2-type cells with an anti-inflammatory phenotype, and the interleukin-10 secreted by them inhibits T-cell proliferation. This immunosuppressive effect related to T-cell proliferation and decrease in cytokine production by MSCs was, among others, confirmed by Sato et al. [85]. However, the mechanisms by which MSCs are mobilized and recruited to damaged sites are not known. In addition, how they survive and differentiate into distinct cell types is still not clear. Once MSCs have been applied to the microenvironment of injured or degenerated tissues, many factors stimulate the release of many growth factors by MSCs; a detailed growth and trophic factor overview is shown in **Table 3**. These growth factors stimulate the development of fibroblasts, endothelial cells, and tissue progenitor cells [86]. It is credible to state that the use of MSCs and their potential in immunomodulation in regenerative medicine applications hold great promise [87].

5.5 MSC growth factor activity

In order for MSCs to differentiate into several cell lineages, the action of specific growth factors and chemical mediators are needed in these processes [88, 89].

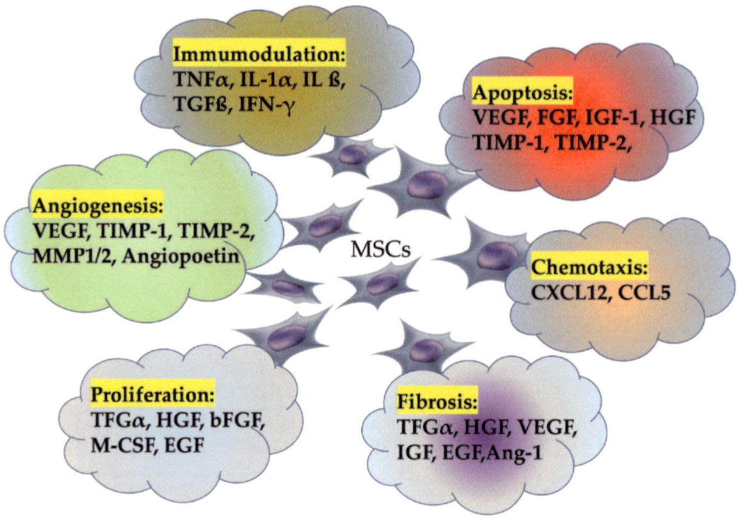

Figure 11.
MSC trophic mechanisms. After bone marrow cell injections, MSCs produce a variety of trophic factors impacting healing cascades by reducing cell apoptosis, fibrosis, and inflammation. Furthermore, by acting on cell proliferation cascades, they contribute to differentiation and mobilization of cells. MSC paracrine trophic factors are potentially important in maintaining endothelial integrity and promoting angiogenesis and the secretion of various growth factors and reparative cytokines.

Growth factor/cytokine	Activity in MSC regenerative repair
Epidermal growth factor	Wound healing
	Tissue regeneration
Fibroblast growth factor	Tissue repair
	Intrinsic stem cell survival
	Tissue regeneration
	Neurogenesis
Hepatocyte growth factor	Vasculogenesis
	Intrinsic neural cell regeneration
Insulin-like growth factor	Wound healing
	Neurogenesis
Keratinocyte growth factor	Wound healing
Platelet-derived growth factor	Tissue repair
Transforming growth factor beta	Wound healing
Vascular endothelial growth factor	Angiogenesis
	Wound healing
Angiopoietin-1	Angiogenesis
	Tissue repair
Erythropoietin	Angiogenesis
Interleukin-8	Wound healing
Stem cell-derived factor-1	Neuroprotective effect
	Wound healing

Table 3.
Growth and trophic factors contributing to MSC tissue regenerative processes.

Once MSCs are mobilized, or after BM tissue injections, they produce a number of trophic factors that impact healing responses. At a local tissue level, they act by reducing cell apoptosis, fibrosis, inflammation, and activation of cascades that lead to cell proliferation and differentiation, mobilization of cells, and an onset of angiogenesis via paracrine and autocrine pathways [90]. Crucial agents involved in these processes include a variety of growth factors. The MSC trophic effects are associated with the secretion of reparative cytokines and growth factors [91], which contribute finally to tissue repair of inflamed and degenerated tissues, retaining positive MSC paracrine effects [92]. Many of the MSC growth factors are generated on the principle of the cell regulating protein nuclear factor-κB activation, after an initial exposure to pro-inflammatory stimuli such as IFN-γ, TNF-α, and IL-1β or even hypoxia [93]. These factors most likely coexist in prepared MSC-containing BM vials and delivered at tissue injury sites. In this situation, MSC growth factors and other cell mediators may have the potential to exert their specific activities via molecular interplays and subsequently promote optimal MSC-associated therapeutic tissue healing, in particular in a highly concentrated environment [94]. The endothelial monolayer barrier function of tissue capillary beds is often disturbed under degenerative and inflamed conditions, allowing for the blood to release proteins and white blood cells, while MSCs produce and release growth factors that affect endothelial cell and subsequently promote the development of tissue progenitor cells and fibroblasts and support tissue regeneration and repair [95]. Some clinicians combine platelet-rich plasma concentrations [96] with BM products in order to have a more biologically active graft, projected to optimize regenerative medicine treatment outcomes. However, it is important to comprehend the detailed mechanisms underlying the inflammation-modulated production of growth factors by MSCs, as this will provide a better perspective for the clinical application of MSCs or their paracrine factors in tissue regeneration.

5.6 MSCs and angiogenesis

MSC paracrine trophic factors are potentially important in maintaining endothelial integrity and promoting angiogenesis through their ability to regulate endothelial cell proliferation and ECM production [97]. Furthermore, endothelial cell permeability is reduced, and MSCs inhibit interactions between leukocytes and endothelial cells [98]. Apart from MSC trophic factors, fibroblasts have fundamental functions in maintaining tissue integrity and promote tissue healing through their secretion of cytokines that support ECM building. These endothelial and angiogenetic capabilities have been demonstrated in clinical studies addressing chronic wound healing [99] and recovery from postmyocardial infarction [100].

5.7 Homing and migration

An enduring problem in the field of cell-based regenerative medicine therapies is the factual delivery of the harvested and prepared cells to the site of injury, a process termed "homing" [101]. One of the major characteristics of MSCs after administration is that they are able to migrate to sites of inflammation and tissue damage, which are typically associated with cytokine outburst [102]. Homing mechanism to degenerated and injured tissue sites are influenced by factors like age, cell viability, the number of available cells (dosage), and the delivery method. Unlike the well-characterized phenomenon of leukocyte homing by de novo, or exogenously delivered (BM) MSCs, is still unclear. Evidently, an increase in leukocyte migration, with induced rolling response to inflamed tissue sites, has been noted by engineered MSCs [103]. For successful cell-based regenerative therapies, it is critically important for MSCs to control cell adhesion in the ECM of the treated tissue. This will occur through the expression of fibronectin and specific integrin and selectin protein adhesion molecules, which are binding to collagen and fibrin ECM components [102], initiating tissue healing and regeneration through cell adhesion, cell growth, migration, and differentiation [104]. The migration ability of MSCs is further controlled by a wide range of growth factors, acting under the receptor tyrosine kinase signaling principle [105], once more illustrating the importance and presence of platelets and their growth factors in the collected BM vial. Furthermore, the administration of MSCs via various delivery routes (intravenous, intraperitoneal, intra-arterial, in situ injections) seems to have an effect on MSC homing [66].

6. Bone marrow aspirate aspiration and processing

When applying regenerative medicine MSC applications, physicians have a choice to use either a BMA as a regenerative injectate, without any processing steps, or they can harvest a particular BMA volume necessary to produce a BMC, with dedicated devices and centrifuges. Additionally, the differences between a BMA injectate only and a BMA concentrate are discussed.

6.1 BMA-MSC procedural steps

In the freshly aspirated BMA samples, the heterogenous cellular content is pervasively distributed in the vial, as long as clotting is prevented.

6.1.1 Anticoagulation protocol

Prior to a BMA procedure, it is recommended that bone marrow harvesting devices, concentration devices, and all of the processing accessories that will be in contact with BM are subject to a thorough heparin rinsing. Furthermore, several instructions for use advice to leave a volume of anticoagulant in the aspiration syringes and processing device as well, as BM tissue has the potential for rapid clotting. Before a BMC concentration device is loaded for processing, the aspiration syringes volumes are transferred into one consolidating collection syringe and subsequently filtered through a 200u heparin rinsed filter to eliminate particles, fibrin strands, and fat tissue.

6.1.2 Two-step BMA centrifugation protocol

It is our belief that the preparation of a vial of concentrated MSCs is best created by the so-called double-spin protocols, using dedicated and approved disposable concentration devices. BMA centrifugal processing techniques, to produce a viable BM-MSC injectate, are generally accepted methods when executed at POC, because these preparation protocols seek to overcome the limitations of MSC ex vivo cell culturing techniques. In this section we touch on a BMC preparation protocol to produce PurePRP SupraPhysiologic Bone Marrow Concentrate (PureBMC®SP, EmCyte Corporation, Fort Myers, FL, USA). The PureBMC®SP autologous biologic is part of an autologous cellular platform technology, facilitating the preparation of platelet-rich plasma and adipose tissue concentrates. A two-step centrifugation and preparation protocol will concentrate the indispensable BMA cellular content to a BMC. Following a first centrifugation spin, the BMA is sequestered in a BM plasma fraction (BMPF), containing a buffy coat layer and RBCs. The BMPF is aspirated, immediately followed by a separate collection of 2 ml of RBCs, following the instructions for use of the PureBMC® concentration device. Both volumes are then transferred for a second centrifugal spin cycle to the concentration compartment of the same device. During the second spin, a specific centrifugation protocol is accomplished, leaving the bone marrow cells in a concentrated fashion attached at the bottom of the chamber. Excessive BMPF is manually removed, leaving behind a specific BMC volume for resuspension. The amount of this volume depends on the requirements for clinical applications. Therefore, the BMC injectate volume may vary between 3 and 10 ml, with increased cell concentrations according to this final volume varying between 4- and 10-fold the native concentrations.

6.2 Cellular differences between BMA and BMC injectates

In a BMA injectate, the concentrations of the cells resemble the concentration of the cells that are present in the bone marrow cavity. However, based on aspiration techniques, the number of MSC might be increased. A BMC is a small volume of fluid containing a high concentration of cells extracted from the bone marrow, such as high yields of MSCs (can be measured as CFU-Fs), HSCs, progenitor cells, total nucleated cells, and platelets, at a significant concentration above BMA baseline values. Furthermore, the heterogenous nature of marrow cells is completed by the presence of increased levels of growth factors [106, 107], cytokines like IL-8, and interleukin-1RA [94]. Additionally, in a BMC injectate following a two-step centrifugation procedure, the RBC and plasma-free hemoglobin (PFH) concentrations are significantly decreased when compared to a BMA injectate.

6.2.1 Red blood cells and hemolysis

Throughout the aspiration procedure, RBCs can be damaged as a result of high shear forces [108]. As a consequence, the RBC membrane will start to disintegrate, and hemolysis, with the release of PFH, will occur. Damaged RBCs and free hemoglobin (Hb) lead to the development and release of toxic Hb forms, like free hemin, ferric Hb, and iron [109]. This is of particular concern as PFH and their split products, heme and iron, cannot be cleared, by natural scavenger proteins, when bone marrow injectates are applied in any microenvironment, as these are outside of the blood stream. A graphic representation of the pathophysiological effects and reactions of PFH, leading to various hemolytic-related sequelae and potentially encumbering clinical outcomes, is presented in **Figure 12**.

6.2.2 Comparative laboratory data BMA vs. BMC

In **Table 1** the effects of concentrating BMA to BMC with regard to some of the most important marrow constituents and factors are shown, as discussed in Section 4.1. The data in the table represent a clinical bilateral BMA model, using two different harvesting systems. For both systems, BMA was aspirated in an identical manner, at three different depth levels collecting in total 10 ml of marrow. Furthermore, to compare the cellular differences between a BMC injectate and a BMA injectate (BMA-MC), we collected an additional 40 ml of BMA with the Aspire system, after the first 10 ml. This allowed for a total processing volume of 60 ml to produce BMC. Laboratory analysis resolved that both BMA devices were almost similar with regard to cell viability and numbers. Interestingly, with regard to CFU-Fs, the data are in accordance with Hernigou [40], and the first marrow aspiration provides the highest number of CFU-Fs. However, when comparing the BMA-MC cellular composition (a patient treatment specimen) with the BMC treatment specimen,

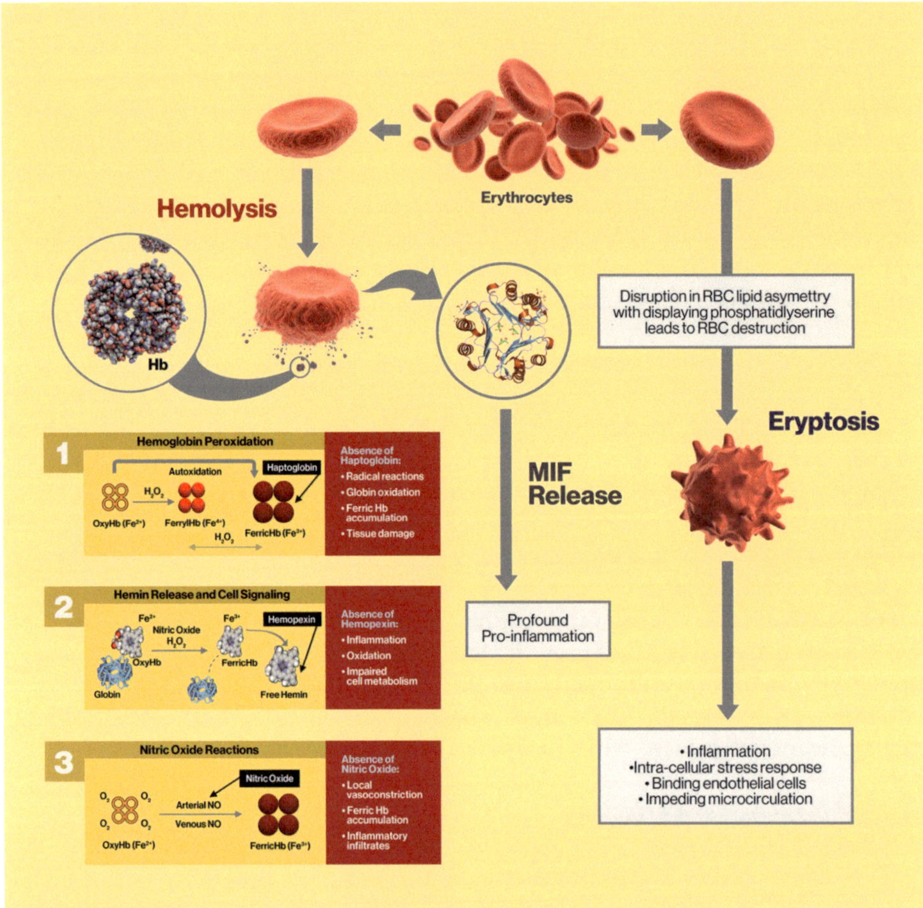

Figure 12.
Pathophysiological effects and reactions of RBCs in BMC vials. In absence of scavengers and compensatory mechanisms, PFH split products can lead to toxic consequences like inflammation and prooxidant effects, endothelial cell dysfunction, and vasoconstriction. Biological treatment specimen, containing high concentrations of RBCs, will lead to RBC cell membrane disruption (eryptosis,) releasing macrophage migration inhibitory factor (MIF) (courtesy of P. Everts and modified from Schaer et al. [109]).

significant differences occur. Centrifugation foremost significantly increases cells who take part in regenerative processes when compared to the BMA-MC product. In contrast the non-regenerative RBCs and PFH concentrations are significantly reduced in the treatment vial, while maintaining a higher cell viability after centrifugation. Our findings, with regard to cellular enrichments comparing a BMA with a BMC, are in agreement with others [41, 110], but not regarding RBC content and PFH. The cell concentrations are not only depending on the centrifugation protocols and the final BMC volume but are contingent of a meticulously executed BMA procedure, maintaining high cell viability, with minimal cell destruction.

6.3 Not every bone marrow concentrate is born equal

Currently, eight BMC harvesting devices are available on the market, producing different formulations of BMC and tissue viabilities and yielding different cellular concentration characteristics [111, 112]. As such, BMC preparations may vary widely regarding HSCs, MSCs, progenitors, platelet growth factors, and RBC content. Given this heterogeneity, the impact of BMC therapies on tissue regeneration may vary greatly. Explicitly, it is important to understand that the BMC non-stem cell cellular components in the treatment vial might have significant roles regarding behavior and function of MSCs. Recently, the cellular variances were confirmed in a systematic review, evaluating BMC studies in musculoskeletal pathologies [53]. Presumably, as postulated by numerous authors, the variances in BMC cellular compositions have a significant effect on the biological activity and regenerative potency of the treatment specimen, and these inconsistencies impact clinical outcomes [111, 113]. Unfortunately, an exact understanding of the underlying signaling relationships is not completely understood [114].

7. Bone marrow-derived mesenchymal cells in musculoskeletal disorders

The use of autologous BM-derived MSCs for the treatment of a variety of musculoskeletal ailments is progressing significantly. Literature findings demonstrate positive outcomes after regenerative medicine MSC applications, in particular in joints, tendons, and bone, and hold great promise for future MSK-D applications, especially if more research and larger clinical trials are performed, focusing on cell validation processes and elucidating on potential dose responses.

7.1 Knee osteoarthritis

In this section we will present several clinical studies in which autologous, heterogenous BMC was used as a regenerative biologic to treat a variety of musculoskeletal disorders [42, 115]. Studies reporting on similar pathologies using BM-derived/cultured MSCs are not mentioned as it has been reported that these technologies have different biomedical properties and extraction methods [116] and potentially possess new challenges and indications, when compared to at POC prepared fresh autologous BMCs. In clinical settings, BMC has been exploited as an ortho-biological treatment option for a range of indications, like symptomatic focal femoral head osteonecrosis, OA of the knee and hip, focal chondral defects, as well as another MSK-D. The rationale to use autologous BMC in osteoarthritic (OA) joints and other indications is its potential in facilitating anti-inflammatory and anabolic effects after injection. Moreover, the heterogenous BMC cellular assortment is known for its angiogenetic properties, therefore contributing to chondrocyte metabolism and inducing homing of (progenitor) stem cells to the treated areas [117]. Rodriguez-Fotan and co-workers used a two-step BMC preparation protocol in patients with early onset of OA in the knee or hip (Kellgren-Lawrence grades I–II, Tönnis grades I–II, respectively), with BMA aspirated from the anterior iliac crest. After a single BMC injection, 63% of treated patients had improved clinical symptoms at 6-month postinjection. They concluded that the intra-articular BMC injections are safe procedures and no adverse events were reported [118]. In a prospective single-blind, placebo-controlled trial, 25 patients with bilateral knee OA and a median age of 60 years were randomized to receive BMC into one knee and saline placebo into the contralateral knee, thereby utilizing each patient as his/her own control. Safety data, effect of pain relief, knee function (Osteoarthritis Research Society International) measures, and the visual analog scale (VAS) for pain were observed until 6 months after the injections [119]. However, no differences between the two groups were observed. Of interest in this study was that the final injectate composition consisted of a mix of BMC and BMPF suspension. However, the eventual consequences of diluting BMC with BMPF on outcomes were not discussed. In another case series by Kim et al., a more invasive treatment approach was used. BMC was mixed with adipose tissue as a multi-tissue preparation for knee OA injections, in patients with a mean age of 60.7 years. At 9-month follow-up, all patients showed clinical improvement, with satisfactory results in 70.7% of patients [120]. Remarkably, the authors found that patients with inferior treatment results had a greater severity of OA prior treatment, as they were marked at Kellgren-Lawrence grade IV, suggesting that advanced OA may be more restrained to BMC therapy. The side effects encountered in this study, joint inflammation and pain, were in accordance with data from Rodriguez-Fotan [118]. Recently, a similar (retrospective) study was executed by Mautner and associates. Patients were prospectively treated either with bone marrow aspirate concentrate (BMAC) or micro-fragmented adipose tissue (MFAT) injections, for symptomatic knee OA [121]. The follow-up responses consisted of 76 patients (with 106 knees). The Knee Injury and Osteoarthritis Outcome Score (KOOS) questionnaire, Emory Quality of Life (EQOL) questionnaire, and VAS for pain were compared with baseline scores for all patients, and outcomes between BMAC and MFAT groups were evaluated. Data demonstrated a significant improvement in joint function and VAS pain scores after both MFAT and BMAC injections. No significant difference between the two autologous biological groups was demonstrating that BM- or adipose tissue-derived ortho-biological injections resulted in similar functional improvements.

7.2 Shoulder disorders

Lately, Darrow et al. reported on patients treated for shoulder osteoarthritis or rotator cuff tears ($N = 50$), with either BMC or BMA injections. Patients were grouped in receiving one or two injections [122]. Outcome reports included resting pain, active pain, upper extremity functionality scale, and overall improvement percentage. Data were compared to baseline and between the two groups. All patients had significant posttreatment improvements in resting pain, active pain, and functionality scores, when compared to baseline values. Patients receiving two treatments, average interval duration of 22 days, experienced statistically significant more improvements in active pain than the patients receiving one injection. There were no significant outcome differences between patients with a rotator cuff tear or OA. Unfortunately, no information was provided on the BMA and BMC procedure, and no laboratory validation data were reported.

7.3 Osteonecrosis

Philippe Hernigou, world renowned for treating femoral head osteonecrosis, advocates the use of autologous BMC cell therapies [123]. He described a substantial repair and stabilization of necrotic femoral heads with percutaneous injection of autologous BMC, in combination with surgical core decompression. In a later paper, he reviews three decades of BMC therapies in hip osteonecrosis, emphasizing the quality of the BMC and cellular competence and addressing the effects of BM cell concentrates on the microenvironmental changes within osteonecrotic bone [124]. Other groups reported on prospective randomized clinical trials for femoral head osteonecrosis, comparing surgical decompression alone versus decompression augmented by autologous BMC preparations. The biologics were implanted during the surgical decompression procedure. In one study, patients were evaluated using the Western Ontario and McMaster Universities Osteoarthritis (WOMAC) Index questionnaire, VAS pain index, and MRI. The mean WOMAC and VAS scores in all patients improved significantly ($P < 0.001$). Post-procedural MRIs showed a significant ($P = 0.046$) improvement in patients in whom the surgical procedure was combined with BMC [125]. In a similar study, a significant decrease in pain associated with a functional benefit lasting the entire observation period was observed in the BMC-treated patients. However, no difference in clinical outcomes between the two study groups was seen during a 2-year follow-up period, with no significant difference between the femoral head survival rate [126]. Importantly, they analyzed the MSC and nuclear cell content of the BMC. There was a significant rise in nuclear cells and CFU-Fs (6.3-fold and 1.5-fold baseline values, respectively). Despite a significant rise in CFU-Fs in the BMC, the total deliverable MSC cell counts were relatively low. This might be related to the design features and specifications of the fully automated, sensor-controlled processing BMC device that was used with a single-step centrifugation protocol.

7.4 Cartilage repair

Awad and associates recently published a meta-analysis on knee cartilage repair [127]. They conducted a systematic review using the PRISMA guidelines and the *Cochrane Handbook for Systematic Reviews of Interventions*. A meta-analysis was conducted to estimate the effect size for function and pain in 724 patients, with a mean age of 44.2 years. In this review, both cultured BM-MSCs and autologous non-cultured BMC were used. All autologous BMC treatment specimens were prepared following a two-step centrifugation method. Their most important meta-analytic finding was that the administration of non-cultured, fresh, BMC significantly reduced pain and improved knee function. This might be induced by the heterogeneous composition of the non-cultured BMC, as all constituents will synergistically foster cartilage regeneration and local pain management. Furthermore, BMC holds a certain volume of autologous plasma which can function as a cellular scaffold with the advantage of a more sustained release, compared to a pure cultured MSC product.

7.5 Tendinopathies

In a retrospective study, Stein et al. used BMC for primary Achilles tendon repairs, following traumatic injuries [128]. The BMC was adjunct to augment the surgical correction. Although the study lacked a control group, at a mean follow-up of 30 months, there were no re-ruptures reported. In a small patient study, centrifuged BMC specimen were injected in patients, refractory to conservative therapies, with clinical and radiological evidence of chronic patellar tendinopathy. Long-term follow-up showed statistically significant improvement in the majority of its reported scores [129]. A series of patients, diagnosed with clinical lateral epicondylitis, were treated with a single-spin BMC protocol. A significant improvement was noted when pre-BMC scores were compared with postinjection scores, at 12-weekpost-intervention. The authors suggested that BMC injections in patients who have failed non-operative treatment, before a surgical intervention, should be considered, and in their belief BMC injections can be developed as second-line conservative treatment in chronic tendinopathy, potentially reversing the degenerative process [130].

8. Bone marrow concentrates in spinal disorders

Degenerative disk disease (DDD) affects the disks that separate the spine bones. Age-related changes can lead to arthritis, disk herniation, or spinal stenosis. Pressure on the spinal cord and nerves may cause pain. DDD is associated with significant morbidity. Conservative treatment options, physical therapy, self-care, medication, and spinal injections are used to manage the symptoms. However, these measures are often not significantly responsive. Surgery has been an option if the pain is chronic. Nowadays, autologous regenerative applications have been made available to patients as an alternative treatment option.

8.1 Degenerative disk disease

Pettine et al. studied the use of intra-discal BMC injections in patients with DDD [131]. The authors injected 26 symptomatic patients for lumbar diskogenic back pain and disability and evaluated their postinjection outcomes using disability scores, pain scores, and MRIs. At 2-year follow-up, patients experienced significant improvements in disability and pain scores. This group was the first to report on MSC dose-dependent outcome responses. Patients receiving greater concentrations of autologous BM-MSC (expressed as CFU-Fs > 2000/ml) experienced a faster and greater reduction in pain scores. Later, these findings were strengthened with a follow-up study at 36 months, showing similar outcome results [43]. At 5-year follow-up, absolute and percentage reductions in pain and disability scores were sustained, with no adverse events reported through the 5-year follow-up period [132]. The American Society of Interventional Pain Physicians published recently guidelines addressing responsible and safe use of autologous biologics in the management of lower back pain [133]. Their extensive analysis revealed that there is level III evidence for the use of PRP and BM-MSCs. The guidelines also state that, following diagnostic evidence, regenerative therapies should be provided to patients as an independent therapy. If appropriate and indicated, regenerative therapies can be combined with conventional medicinal therapy or in conjunction with physical and behavioral therapy.

8.2 Spinal surgery

Hart et al. informed on a prospective, randomized, and blinded study in patients with lumbar disease the use of BMC mixed with allograft spongiosa chips during surgical posterolateral fusion (PLF) procedures. Patients underwent instrumented lumbar spine PLF procedures [134]. Fusion status and the degree of mineralization were evaluated by two radiologists blinded to patient group affiliation. X-ray examination, in control patients at 12-month follow-up, showed that the bone graft mass fused in none of the cases and, at 24-months, in four cases (10%). In the BMC treatment group, 6 cases (15%) achieved fusion at 12 months and 14 cases (35%) at 24 months. Computed tomography scans showed that 40% of control patients and 80% of BMC-treated patients had evidence of at least a unilateral continuous bridging of the bones between neighboring vertebrae at 24 months, significantly favoring the mixture of spongiosa bone with autologous BMC ($P < 0.05$) as an efficient option to augment PLF healing.

9. Bone marrow concentrates in chronic wounds

Cell-based therapies are an attractive approach for the treatment of recalcitrant chronic wounds. BM-MSCs have been studied as a therapeutic strategy in chronic hard-to-heal wounds [135]. The orchestrated process of wound healing entails cellular and hormonal physiological processes in inflammation, proliferation, collagen matrix formation, and epithelialization which are regulated by various platelet-derived growth factors, such as TGF-b, VEGF, PDGF, granulocyte-macrophage colony-stimulating factor, the interleukin family, EGF, FGF, and TNF-a [44, 105]. In chronic, poor-healing wounds, the activity and effectivity of growth factors and cytokines are often reduced due to a chronically inflamed wound.

Under these conditions the neo-angiogenetic wound healing potential is reduced, resulting in poor or no full wound epithelialization. The rationale for using BMC in these patients is the potential to modulate the immune response and secreting paracrine factors which promote (neo) angiogenesis, thereby providing biological ingredients for wound tissue repair that can jumpstart full wound closure [76, 136]. Optimal wound bed preparation is of the essence in wound healing strategies and encompasses tissue debridement with proper management of the bacterial load. Based on BM-MSC characteristics and their biological activity, MSCs are capable of interacting with resident wound cells to transform resident cells to functional matrix building cells, as described by Balaji et al. [137]. This finding might be of particular importance for dermal rebuilding processes, to stimulate (transplanted) keratinocyte-mediated wound epithelialization.

10. Bone marrow concentrates in critical limb ischemia

Patients with significant, below the knee, vascular diseases and who are, first of all, not eligible for revascularization surgery or endovascular treatments due to several comorbidities or have high operative risk and had multiple failures of revascularization or high rate of re-stenosis, might be suitable candidates for biological cell-based therapy with BM-MSCs. Patients diagnosed with critical limb ischemia (CLI) might also suffer from chronic non-healing wounds, and the estimated amputation and mortality rates are high [138]. The application of regenerative medicine therapies, in particular the use of BM-MSCs protocols, has merged as a treatment option in patients with CLI. In these patients, the justification to use BMC is to promote the regeneration of impaired endothelium and stimulate neo-angiogenesis in ischemic areas [139]. Several varieties of BM-MSC therapies have been studied in CLI patients, ranging from BM-derived mononuclear cells, CD34+ BM cells, to mesenchymal stromal cells. The outcomes of cell-based trials have been encouraging and demonstrated a significant decrease in the rate of amputation [140]. It can be concluded that BM-MSC applications have the potential to modify the natural history of intractable CLI, while high-quality randomized trials are needed [45].

11. Conclusions

Regenerative medicine technologies offer solutions to a number of compelling clinical problems that have not been able to adequately result in a solution through the use of drugs, surgery, or permanent replacement devices. Reviewing the last decades regarding autologous biological therapies, BM-MSCs have gained great interest. The purpose of this chapter was to review specific characteristics of bone marrow tissue and its cellular content, in particular the mesenchymal stem cells. Considerations when performing aspiration techniques and bone marrow concentrate preparations were presented, including explicit roles of hematopoietic and mesenchymal stem cells and other cytokines. Among autologous tissue-based cellular therapies, bone marrow mesenchymal cell therapies have been the most frequently employed and reported on, despite the fact that effects of coadjuvants, dosing, repetitive procedures, etc. are not yet established. Cultured MSC therapeutic interventions require strict procedures and biological license agreements, making them less attractive for same-day regenerative therapies. Using at POC BM-MSC concentrates overcomes these lengthy regulatory processes without the need for mandates. Clinical translation of BM-MSC-based therapies remains a work in progress, as proper standardization has not yet been recognized [53]. However, in the clinical setting, effective and safe autologous BMA harvesting and preparation of BMC have been reported [42]. More, better, organized randomized clinical trials that are warranted with accurate follow-up data revealing the efficacy of BM-MSC therapy, including laboratory validation of the used products, should be a future goal. Furthermore, proper deliberations should manage the enormous variability aspects, like aspiration techniques, imaging options and procedures, BMC preparation protocols, effect of patient age, as well as tissue disease state. Therapy failures should also be highlighted in order to understand how they impact the therapy outcomes. Ultimately, the adoption of an accepted standard of overall regenerative biological preparations, including critical and ambivalent nuances, is crucial for future regenerative medicine practices.

Conflict of interest

Author P. Everts is also the chief scientific officer of the EmCyte Corporation.

Author details

Peter A. Everts[1*], Glenn Flanagan II[2], Joshua Rothenberg[3] and Kenneth Mautner[4]

1 Scientific and Educational Division, Gulf Coast Biologics, Fort Myers, FL, USA

2 Naples Regenerative Institute, Regenerative Orthopedics Interventional Spine and Joint, Naples, FL, USA

3 Boca Raton Regional Hospital and Baptist Health South Florida, Regenerative Medicine and Boca Care Orthopedics and Interventional Sports and Spine, Deerfield Beach, FL, USA

4 Emory Sports Medicine and Primary Care Sports Medicine, Emory University, Atlanta, GA, USA

*Address all correspondence to: peter@gulfcoastbiologics.com

References

[1] Becker AJ, McCulloch EA, Till JE. Cytological demonstration of the clonal nature of spleen colonies derived from transplanted mouse marrow cells. Nature. 1963;**197**(4866):452-454

[2] Lee EH, Hui JHP. The potential of stem cells in orthopaedic surgery. Journal of Bone and Joint Surgery. 2006;**88**(7):11

[3] Jing B, Yuan H, Yi-Ru W, Li-Feng L, Jie C, Shao-Ping S, et al. Comparison of human amniotic fluid-derived and umbilical cord Wharton's Jelly-derived mesenchymal stromal cells: Characterization and myocardial differentiation capacity: Comparison of human amniotic fluid-derived and umbilical cord Wharton's Jelly-derived mesenchymal stromal cells: Characterization and myocardial differentiation capacity. Journal of Geriatric Cardiology. 2012;**9**(2):166-171

[4] Charbord P. Bone marrow mesenchymal stem cells: Historical overview and concepts. Human Gene Therapy. 2010;**21**(9):1045-1056

[5] Caplan AI. Mesenchymal stem cells. Journal of Orthopaedic Research. 1991;**9**(5):641-650

[6] Samsonraj RM, Raghunath M, Nurcombe V, Hui JH, van Wijnen AJ, Cool SM. Concise review: Multifaceted characterization of human mesenchymal stem cells for use in regenerative medicine: Characterization of human mesenchymal stem cells. Stem Cells Translational Medicine. 2017;**6**(12):2173-2185

[7] Pittenger MF. Multilineage potential of adult human mesenchymal stem cells. Science. 1999;**284**(5411):143-147

[8] Hernández-Gil IF-T, Gracia MAA, Jerez B. Physiological bases of bone regeneration I. Histology and physiology of bone tissue. Medicina Oral, Patología Oral y Cirugía Bucal. 2006;**11**:E47-E51

[9] Kopp H-G, Avecilla ST, Hooper AT, Rafii S. The bone marrow vascular niche: Home of HSC differentiation and mobilization. Physiology. 2005;**20**(5):349-356

[10] McDaniel JS, Antebi B, Pilia M, Hurtgen BJ, Belenkiy S, Necsoiu C, et al. Quantitative assessment of optimal bone marrow site for the isolation of porcine mesenchymal stem cells. Stem Cells International. 2017;**2017**:1-10

[11] Gurevitch O, Slavin S, Feldman AG. Conversion of red bone marrow into yellow—Cause and mechanisms. Medical Hypotheses. 2007;**69**(3):531-536

[12] Bonomo A, Monteiro AC, Gonçalves-Silva T, Cordeiro-Spinetti E, Galvani RG, Balduino A. A T cell view of the bone marrow. Frontiers in Immunology. 2016;**7**:194. DOI: 10.3389/fimmu.2016.00184

[13] Lambertsen H. Study of the distribution marrow colonies. Blood. 1984;**63**:287-297

[14] Muguruma Y, Yahata T, Miyatake H, Sato T, Uno T, Itoh J, et al. Reconstitution of the functional human hematopoietic microenvironment derived from human mesenchymal stem cells in the murine bone marrow compartment. Blood. 2006;**107**(5):1878-1887

[15] Fliedner TM, Graessle D, Paulsen C, Reimers K. Structure and function of bone marrow hemopoiesis: Mechanisms of response to ionizing radiation exposure. Cancer Biotherapy & Radiopharmaceuticals. 2002;**17**(4):405-426

[16] Rafii S, Lyden D. Therapeutic stem and progenitor cell transplantation for

organ vascularization and regeneration. Nature Medicine. 2003;**9**(6):11

[17] Spradling A, Drummond-Barbosa D, Kai T. Stem cells find their niche. Nature. 2001;**414**(6859):98-104

[18] Li L, Xie T. Stem cell niche: Structure and function. The Annual Review of Cell and Developmental Biology. 2005;**21**:605-631

[19] Ehninger A, Trumpp A. The bone marrow stem cell niche grows up: Mesenchymal stem cells and macrophages move in. The Journal of Experimental Medicine. 2011;**208**(3):421-428

[20] Wu P, Tarasenko YI, Gu Y, Huang L-YM, Coggeshall RE, Yu Y. Region-specific generation of cholinergic neurons from fetal human neural stem cells grafted in adult rat. Nature Neuroscience. 2002;**5**(12):1271-1278

[21] Zhao L-R, Duan W-M, Reyes M, Keene CD, Verfaillie CM, Low WC. Human bone marrow stem cells exhibit neural phenotypes and ameliorate neurological deficits after grafting into the ischemic brain of rats. Experimental Neurology. 2002;**174**(1):11-20

[22] Morrison SJ, Scadden DT. The bone marrow niche for haematopoietic stem cells. Nature. 2014;**505**(7483):327-334

[23] Schofield R. The relationship between the spleen colony-forming cell and the haemopoietic stem cell. Blood Cells. 1978;**4**(1-2):7-25

[24] Krebsbach PH, Kuznetsov SA, Bianco P, Gehron RP. Bone marrow stromal cells: Characterization and clinical application. Critical Reviews in Oral Biology and Medicine. 1999;**10**(2):165-181

[25] Yin T. The stem cell niches in bone. The Journal of Clinical Investigation. 2006;**116**(5):1195-1201

[26] Calvi LM, Link DC. The hematopoietic stem cell niche in homeostasis and disease. Blood. 2015;**126**(22):2443-2451

[27] Kiel MJ, Radice GL, Morrison SJ. Lack of evidence that hematopoietic stem cells depend on N-cadherin-mediated adhesion to osteoblasts for their maintenance. Cell Stem Cell. 2007;**1**(2):204-217

[28] Anthony BA, Link DC. Regulation of hematopoietic stem cells by bone marrow stromal cells. Trends in Immunology. 2014;**35**(1):32-37

[29] Nombela-Arrieta C, Pivarnik G, Winkel B, Canty KJ, Harley B, Mahoney JE, et al. Quantitative imaging of haematopoietic stem and progenitor cell localization and hypoxic status in the bone marrow microenvironment. Nature Cell Biology. 2013;**15**(5):533-543

[30] Sacchetti B, Funari A, Michienzi S, Di Cesare S, Piersanti S, Saggio I, et al. Self-renewing osteoprogenitors in bone marrow sinusoids can organize a hematopoietic microenvironment. Cell. 2007;**131**(2):324-336

[31] Shi S, Gronthos S. Perivascular niche of postnatal mesenchymal stem cells in human bone marrow and dental pulp. Journal of Bone and Mineral Research. 2003;**18**(4):696-704

[32] Méndez-Ferrer S, Lucas D, Battista M, Frenette PS. Haematopoietic stem cell release is regulated by circadian oscillations. Nature. 2008;**452**(7186):442-447

[33] Kunisaki Y, Bruns I, Scheiermann C, Ahmed J, Pinho S, Zhang D, et al. Arteriolar niches maintain haematopoietic stem cell quiescence. Nature. 2013;**502**(7473):637-643

[34] Caplan AI. New MSC: MSCs as pericytes are sentinels and

gatekeepers: MSCs, pericytes, metastasis, regenerative mediine. Journal of Orthopaedic Research. 2017;**35**(6):1151-1159

[35] Zhao M, Perry JM, Marshall H, Venkatraman A, Qian P, He XC, et al. Megakaryocytes maintain homeostatic quiescence and promote post-injury regeneration of hematopoietic stem cells. Nature Medicine. 2014;**20**(11):1321-1326

[36] Discher DE, Mooney DJ, Zandstra PW. Growth factors, matrices, and forces combine and control stem cells. Science. 2009;**324**(5935):1673-1677

[37] Chung C, Burdick JA. Influence of three-dimensional hyaluronic acid microenvironments on mesenchymal stem cell Chondrogenesis. Tissue Engineering. Part A. 2009;**15**(2):243-254

[38] Djouad F, Delorme B, Maurice M, Bony C, Apparailly F, Louis-Plence P, et al. Microenvironmental changes during differentiation of mesenchymal stem cells towards chondrocytes. Arthritis Research & Therapy. 2007;**9**(2):R33

[39] Kolf CM, Cho E, Tuan RS. Mesenchymal stromal cells biology of adult mesenchymal stem cells: Regulation of niche, self-renewal and differentiation. Arthritis Research & Therapy. 2007;**9**(1):204

[40] Hernigou P, Homma Y, Flouzat Lachaniette CH, Poignard A, Allain J, Chevallier N, et al. Benefits of small volume and small syringe for bone marrow aspirations of mesenchymal stem cells. International Orthopaedics. 2013;**37**(11):2279-2287

[41] Oliver K, Awan T, Bayes M. Single- versus multiple-site harvesting techniques for bone marrow concentrate: Evaluation of aspirate quality and pain. Orthopaedic Journal of Sports Medicine. 2017;**5**(8):232596711772439

[42] Imam MA, Mahmoud SSS, Holton J, Abouelmaati D, Elsherbini Y, Snow M. A systematic review of the concept and clinical applications of bone marrow aspirate concentrate in orthopaedics. SICOT Journal. 2017;**3**:17

[43] Pettine KA, Suzuki RK, Sand TT, Murphy MB. Autologous bone marrow concentrate intradiscal injection for the treatment of degenerative disc disease with three-year follow-up. International Orthopaedics. 2017;**41**(10):2097-2103

[44] Everts PA. Autologous platelet-rich plasma and mesenchymal stem cells for the treatment of chronic wounds. In: Hakan Dogan K, editor. Wound Healing—Current Perspectives [Internet]. Rijeka: IntechOpen; 2019. Available from: https://www.intechopen.com/books/wound-healing-current-perspectives/autologous-platelet-rich-plasma-and-mesenchymal-stem-cells-for-the-treatment-of-chronic-wounds [Accessed: 4 October 2019]

[45] Pignon B, Sevestre M-A, Kanagaratnam L, Pernod G, Stephan D, Emmerich J, et al. Autologous bone marrow mononuclear cell implantation and its impact on the outcome of patients with critical limb ischemia—Results of a randomized, double-blind, placebo-controlled trial. Circulation Journal. 2017;**81**(11):1713-1720

[46] Lee S-H, Erber WN, Porwit A, Tomonaga M, Peterson LC, International Council for Standardization in Hematology. ICSH guidelines for the standardization of bone marrow specimens and reports. International Journal of Laboratory Hematology. 2008;**30**(5):349-364

[47] Scarpone M, Kuebler D, Chambers A, De Filippo CM, Amatuzio M, Ichim TE, et al. Isolation

of clinically relevant concentrations of bone marrow mesenchymal stem cells without centrifugation. Journal of Translational Medicine. 2019;**17**(1):10

[48] Batinić D, Marusić M, Pavletić Z, Bogdanić V, Uzarević B, Nemet D, et al. Relationship between differing volumes of bone marrow aspirates and their cellular composition. Bone Marrow Transplantation. 1990;**6**(2):103-107

[49] Haseler LJ, Sibbitt RR, Sibbitt WL, Michael AA, Gasparovic CM, Bankhurst AD. Syringe and needle size, syringe type, vacuum generation, and needle control in aspiration procedures. Cardiovascular and Interventional Radiology. 2011;**34**(3):590-600

[50] Friedlis MF, Centeno CJ. Performing a better bone marrow aspiration. Physical Medicine and Rehabilitation Clinics of North America. 2016;**27**(4):919-939

[51] Hirahara AM, Panero A, Andersen WJ. An MRI analysis of the pelvis to determine the ideal method for ultrasound-guided bone marrow aspiration from the iliac crest. American Journal of Orthopedics (Belle Mead, NJ) [Internet]. 2018;**47**(5). DOI: 10.12788/ajo.2018.0038

[52] Hernigou J, Alves A, Homma Y, Guissou I, Hernigou P. Anatomy of the ilium for bone marrow aspiration: Map of sectors and implication for safe trocar placement. International Orthopaedics. 2014;**38**(12):2585-2590

[53] Murray IR, Robinson PG, West CC, Goudie EB, Yong LY, White TO, et al. Reporting standards in clinical studies evaluating bone marrow aspirate concentrate: A systematic review. Arthroscopy: The Journal of Arthroscopic & Related Surgery. 2018;**34**(4):1366-1375

[54] Marx RE, Tursun R. A qualitative and quantitative analysis of autologous human multipotent adult stem cells derived from three anatomic areas by marrow aspiration: Tibia, anterior ilium, and posterior ilium. The International Journal of Oral & Maxillofacial Implants. 2013;**28**(5):e290-e294

[55] Narbona-Carceles J, Vaquero J, Suárez-Sancho S, Forriol F, Fernández-Santos ME. Bone marrow mesenchymal stem cell aspirates from alternative sources is the knee as good as the iliac crest? Injury. 2014;**45**:S42-S47

[56] Chotinantakul K, Leeanansaksiri W. Hematopoietic stem cell development, niches, and signaling pathways. Bone Marrow Research. 2012;**2012**:1-16

[57] Catlin SN, Busque L, Gale RE, Guttorp P, Abkowitz JL. The replication rate of human hematopoietic stem cells in vivo. Blood. 2011;**117**(17):4460-4466

[58] Nygren JM, Jovinge S, Breitbach M, Säwén P, Röll W, Hescheler J, et al. Bone marrow-derived hematopoietic cells generate cardiomyocytes at a low frequency through cell fusion, but not transdifferentiation. Nature Medicine. 2004;**10**(5):494-501

[59] Yancopoulos GD, Davis S, Gale NW, Rudge JS, Wiegand SJ, Holash J. Vascular-specific growth factors and blood vessel formation. Nature. 2000;**407**(6801):242-248

[60] Patel DM, Shah J, Srivastava AS. Therapeutic potential of mesenchymal stem cells in regenerative medicine. Stem Cells International. 2013;**2013**:1-15

[61] Granero-Molto F, Weis JA, Longobardi L, Spagnoli A. Role of mesenchymal stem cells in regenerative medicine: Application to bone and cartilage repair. Expert Opinion on Biological Therapy. 2008;**8**(3):255-268

[62] Oh M, Nör JE. The perivascular niche and self-renewal of stem cells.

Frontiers in Physiology. 2015;**6**:367. DOI: 10.3389/fphys.2015.00367

[63] Rodini CO, da Silva PBG, Assoni AF, Carvalho VM, Okamoto OK. Mesenchymal stem cells enhance tumorigenic properties of human glioblastoma through independent cell–cell communication mechanisms. Oncotarget [Internet]. 2018;**3**

[64] Neri S. Genetic stability of mesenchymal stromal cells for regenerative medicine applications: A fundamental biosafety aspect. International Journal of Molecular Sciences. 2019;**20**(10):2406

[65] Lohan P, Coleman CM, Murphy J, Griffin MD, Ritter T, Ryan AE. Changes in immunological profile of allogeneic mesenchymal stem cells after differentiation: Should we be concerned? Stem Cell Research & Therapy. 2014;**5**(4):99

[66] Karp JM, Leng Teo GS. Mesenchymal stem cell homing: The devil is in the details. Cell Stem Cell. 2009;**4**(3):206-216

[67] Rombouts WJC, Ploemacher RE. Primary murine MSC show highly efficient homing to the bone marrow but lose homing ability following culture. Leukemia. 2003;**17**(1):160-170

[68] LaPrade RF, Dragoo JL, Koh JL, Murray IR, Geeslin AG, Chu CR. AAOS research symposium updates and consensus: Biologic treatment of orthopaedic injuries. The Journal of the American Academy of Orthopaedic Surgeons. 2016;**24**(7):e62-e78

[69] Dominici M, Le Blanc K, Mueller I, Slaper-Cortenbach I, Marini FC, Krause DS, et al. Minimal criteria for defining multipotent mesenchymal stromal cells. The International Society for Cellular Therapy position statement. Cytotherapy. 2006;**8**(4):315-317

[70] Ikebe C, Suzuki K. Mesenchymal stem cells for regenerative therapy: Optimization of cell preparation protocols. BioMed Research International. 2014;**2014**:1-11

[71] Morita Y, Ema H, Nakauchi H. Heterogeneity and hierarchy within the most primitive hematopoietic stem cell compartment. The Journal of Experimental Medicine. 2010;**207**(6):1173-1182

[72] Fellows CR, Matta C, Zakany R, Khan IM, Mobasheri A. Adipose, bone marrow and synovial joint-derived mesenchymal stem cells for cartilage repair. Frontiers in Genetics. 2016;**7**:213. DOI: 10.3389/fgene.2016.00213

[73] Colter DC, Sekiya I, Prockop DJ. Identification of a subpopulation of rapidly self-renewing and multipotential adult stem cells in colonies of human marrow stromal cells. Proceedings of the National Academy of Sciences. 2001;**98**(14):7841-7845

[74] Gothard D, Dawson JI, Oreffo ROC. Assessing the potential of colony morphology for dissecting the CFU-F population from human bone marrow stromal cells. Cell and Tissue Research. 2013;**352**(2):237-247

[75] Cucchiarini M, Venkatesan JK, Ekici M, Schmitt G, Madry H. Human mesenchymal stem cells overexpressing therapeutic genes: From basic science to clinical applications for articular cartilage repair. Bio-Medical Materials and Engineering. 2012;**4**:197-208

[76] Badiavas EV. Treatment of chronic wounds with bone marrow–derived cells. Archives of Dermatology. 2003;**139**(4):510

[77] da Silva ML, Fontes AM, Covas DT, Caplan AI. Mechanisms involved in the therapeutic properties of mesenchymal

stem cells. Cytokine & Growth Factor Reviews. 2009;**20**(5-6):419-427

[78] Bashir J, Sherman A, Lee H, Kaplan L, Hare JM. Mesenchymal stem cell therapies in the treatment of musculoskeletal diseases. Physical Medicine and Rehabilitation. 2014;**6**(1):61-69

[79] Caplan A. Why are MSCs therapeutic? New data: New insight. The Journal of Pathology. 2009;**217**(2):318-324

[80] Siegel G, Schäfer R, Dazzi F. The immunosuppressive properties of mesenchymal stem cells. Transplantation. 2009;**87**(Suppl):S45-S49

[81] Cassatella MA, Mosna F, Micheletti A, Lisi V, Tamassia N, Cont C, et al. Toll-like receptor-3-activated human mesenchymal stromal cells significantly prolong the survival and function of neutrophils. Stem Cells. 2011;**29**(6):1001-1011

[82] Moll G, Jitschin R, von Bahr L, Rasmusson-Duprez I, Sundberg B, Lönnies L, et al. Mesenchymal stromal cells engage complement and complement receptor bearing innate effector cells to modulate immune responses. PLoS One. 2011;**6**(7):e21703

[83] Brandau S, Jakob M, Bruderek K, Bootz F, Giebel B, Radtke S, et al. Mesenchymal stem cells augment the anti-bacterial activity of neutrophil granulocytes. PLoS One. 2014;**9**(9):e106903

[84] Jiang X-X, Zhang Y, Liu B, Zhang S-X, Wu Y, Yu X-D, et al. Human mesenchymal stem cells inhibit differentiation and function of monocyte-derived dendritic cells. Blood. 2005;**105**(10):4120-4126

[85] Sato K, Ozaki K, Oh I, Meguro A, Hatanaka K, Nagai T, et al. Nitric oxide plays a critical role in suppression of T-cell proliferation by mesenchymal stem cells. Blood. 2007;**109**(1):228-234

[86] Shi Y et al. Mesenchymal stem cells a new strategy for immunosuppression and tissue repair. Cell Research. 2010;**20**:510-518

[87] Li W, Ren G, Huang Y, Su J, Han Y, Li J, et al. Mesenchymal stem cells: A double-edged sword in regulating immune responses. Cell Death and Differentiation. 2012;**19**(9):1505-1513

[88] Zisa D, Shabbir A, Suzuki G, Lee T. Vascular endothelial growth factor (VEGF) as a key therapeutic trophic factor in bone marrow mesenchymal stem cell-mediated cardiac repair. Biochemical and Biophysical Research Communications. 2009;**390**(3):834-838

[89] Park JS, Chu JS, Tsou AD, Diop R, Tang Z, Wang A, et al. The effect of matrix stiffness on the differentiation of mesenchymal stem cells in response to TGF-β. Biomaterials. 2011;**32**(16):3921-3930

[90] Caplan AI, Dennis JE. Mesenchymal stem cells as trophic mediators. Journal of Cellular Biochemistry. 2006;**98**(5):1076-1084

[91] Caplan AI, Correa D. The MSC: An injury drugstore. Cell Stem Cell. 2011;**9**(1):11-15

[92] English K. Mechanisms of mesenchymal stromal cell immunomodulation. Immunology and Cell Biology. 2013;**91**(1):19-26

[93] Crisostomo PR, Wang Y, Markel TA, Wang M, Lahm T, Meldrum DR. Human mesenchymal stem cells stimulated by TNF-alpha, LPS, or hypoxia produce growth factors by an NFκB- but not JNK-dependent mechanism. The American Journal of Physiology-Cell Physiology. 2008;**294**:8

[94] Cassano JM, Kennedy JG, Ross KA, Fraser EJ, Goodale MB, Fortier LA. Bone marrow concentrate and platelet-rich plasma differ in cell distribution and interleukin 1 receptor antagonist protein concentration. Knee Surgery, Sports Traumatology, Arthroscopy. 2018;**26**(1):333-342

[95] Ma S, Xie N, Li W, Yuan B, Shi Y, Wang Y. Immunobiology of mesenchymal stem cells. Cell Death and Differentiation. 2014;**21**(2):216-225

[96] Everts PA, Overdevest EP, Jakimowicz JJ, Oosterbos CJ, Schönberger JP, Knape JT, et al. The use of autologous platelet–leukocyte gels to enhance the healing process in surgery, a review. Surgical Endoscopy. 2007;**21**(11):2063-2068

[97] Lee JW, Fang X, Krasnodembskaya A, Howard JP, Matthay MA. Concise review: mesenchymal stem cells for acute lung injury: Role of paracrine soluble factors. Stem Cells. 2011;**29**(6):913-919

[98] Giacca M, Zacchigna S. VEGF gene therapy: Therapeutic angiogenesis in the clinic and beyond. Gene Therapy. 2012;**19**(6):622-629

[99] Chen L, Tredget EE, Wu PYG, Wu Y. Paracrine factors of mesenchymal stem cells recruit macrophages and endothelial lineage cells and enhance wound healing. PLoS One. 2008;**3**(4):e1886

[100] Timmers L, Lim SK, Hoefer IE, Arslan F, Lai RC, van Oorschot AAM, et al. Human mesenchymal stem cell-conditioned medium improves cardiac function following myocardial infarction. Stem Cell Research. 2011;**6**(3):206-214

[101] Sohni A, Verfaillie CM. Mesenchymal stem cells migration homing and tracking. Stem Cells International. 2013;**2013**:1-8

[102] Eggenhofer E, Luk F, Dahlke MH, Hoogduijn MJ. The life and fate of mesenchymal stem cells. Frontiers in Immunology. 2014;**5**:148. DOI: 10.3389/fimmu.2014.00148

[103] Sarkar D, Vemula PK, Zhao W, Gupta A, Karnik R, Karp JM. Engineered mesenchymal stem cells with self-assembled vesicles for systemic cell targeting. Biomaterials. 2010;**31**(19):5266-5274

[104] Midwood KS, Mao Y, Hsia HC, Valenick LV, Schwarzbauer JE. Modulation of cell–fibronectin matrix interactions during tissue repair. The Journal of Investigative Dermatology. Symposium Proceedings. 2006;**11**(1):73-78

[105] Everts PAM, Knape JTA, Weibrich G, Hoffmann J, Overdevest EP, Box HAM, et al. Platelet-rich plasma and platelet gel: A review. The Journal of Extra-Corporeal Technology. 2007;**14**:174-184

[106] Sugaya H, Yoshioka T, Kato T, Taniguchi Y, Kumagai H, Hyodo K, et al. Comparative analysis of cellular and growth factor composition in bone marrow aspirate concentrate and platelet-rich Plasma. Bone Marrow Research. 2018;**2018**:1-9

[107] Piuzzi NS, Khlopas A, Newman JM, Ng M, Roche M, Husni ME, et al. Bone marrow cellular therapies: Novel therapy for knee osteoarthritis. The Journal of Knee Surgery. 2018;**31**(1):22-26

[108] Everts PA, Malanga GA, Paul RV, Rothenberg JB, Stephens N, Mautner KR. Assessing clinical implications and perspectives of the pathophysiological effects of erythrocytes and plasma free hemoglobin in autologous biologics for use in musculoskeletal regenerative medicine therapies. A review. Regenerative Therapy. 2019;**11**:56-64

[109] Schaer DJ, Buehler PW, Alayash AI, Belcher JD, Vercellotti GM. Hemolysis and free hemoglobin revisited: Exploring hemoglobin and hemin scavengers as a novel class of therapeutic proteins. Blood. 2013;**121**(8):1276-1284

[110] Jäger M, Herten M, Fochtmann U, Fischer J, Hernigou P, Zilkens C, et al. Bridging the gap: Bone marrow aspiration concentrate reduces autologous bone grafting in osseous defects. Journal of Orthopaedic Research. 2011;**29**(2):173-180

[111] Hegde V, Shonuga O, Ellis S, Fragomen A, Kennedy J, Kudryashov V, et al. A prospective comparison of 3 approved systems for autologous bone marrow concentration demonstrated nonequivalency in progenitor cell number and concentration. Journal of Orthopaedic Trauma. 2014;**28**(10):591-598

[112] Gaul F, Bugbee WD, Hoenecke HR, D'Lima DD. A review of commercially available point-of-care devices to concentrate bone marrow for the treatment of osteoarthritis and focal cartilage lesions. Cartilage. 2019;**10**(4):387-394

[113] Centeno CJ, Al-Sayegh H, Bashir J, Goodyear S, Freeman MD. A dose response analysis of a specific bone marrow concentrate treatment protocol for knee osteoarthritis. BMC Musculoskeletal Disorders. 2015;**16**(1):258

[114] Murray IR, West CC, Hardy WR, James AW, Park TS, Nguyen A, et al. Natural history of mesenchymal stem cells, from vessel walls to culture vessels. Cellular and Molecular Life Sciences. 2014;**71**(8):1353-1374

[115] Piuzzi NS, Hussain ZB, Chahla J, Cinque ME, Moatshe G, Mantripragada VP, et al. Variability in the preparation, reporting, and use of bone marrow aspirate concentrate in musculoskeletal disorders: A systematic review of the clinical orthopaedic literature. Journal of Bone and Joint Surgery. 2018;**100**(6):517-525

[116] Centeno CJ, Hyzy MW, Williams CJ. Bone marrow derived stem cells and their application in pain medicine. In: Diwan S, Deer TR, editors. Advanced Procedures for Pain Management: A Step-by-Step Atlas [Internet]. Cham: Springer International Publishing; 2018. pp. 469-487. DOI: 10.1007/978-3-319-68841-1_40

[117] Holton J, Imam M, Ward J, Snow M. The basic science of bone marrow aspirate concentrate in chondral injuries. Orthopedic Reviews. 2016;**8**:80-84

[118] Rodriguez-Fontan F, Piuzzi NS, Kraeutler MJ, Pascual-Garrido C. Early clinical outcomes of intra-articular injections of bone marrow aspirate concentrate for the treatment of early osteoarthritis of the hip and knee: A cohort study. Physical Medicine and Rehabilitation. 2018;**10**(12):1353-1359

[119] Shapiro SA, Kazmerchak SE, Heckman MG, Zubair AC, O'Connor MI. A prospective, single-blind, placebo-controlled trial of bone marrow aspirate concentrate for knee osteoarthritis. The American Journal of Sports Medicine. 2017;**45**(1):82-90

[120] Kim J-D, Lee GW, Jung GH, Kim CK, Kim T, Park JH, et al. Clinical outcome of autologous bone marrow aspirates concentrate (BMAC) injection in degenerative arthritis of the knee. European Journal of Orthopaedic Surgery and Traumatology. 2014;**24**(8):1505-1511

[121] Mautner K, Bowers R, Easley K, Fausel Z, Robinson R. Functional outcomes following microfragmented adipose tissue versus bone marrow aspirate concentrate injections for symptomatic knee osteoarthritis.

Stem Cells Translational Medicine. 2019;**8**(11):1149-1156

[122] Darrow M, Shaw B, Schmidt N, Boeger G, Budgett S. Treatment of shoulder osteoarthritis and rotator cuff tears with bone marrow concentrate and whole bone marrow injections. Cogent Medicine. 2019;**6**:1628883. DOI: 10.1080/2331205X.2019.1628883

[123] Hernigou P, Flouzat-Lachaniette C-H, Delambre J, Poignard A, Allain J, Chevallier N, et al. Osteonecrosis repair with bone marrow cell therapies: State of the clinical art. Bone. 2015;**70**:102-109

[124] Hernigou P, Daltro G, Hernigou J. Hip osteonecrosis: Stem cells for life or behead and arthroplasty? International Orthopaedics. 2018;**42**(7):1425-1428

[125] Tabatabaee RM, Saberi S, Parvizi J, Mortazavi SMJ, Farzan M. Combining concentrated autologous bone marrow stem cells injection with core decompression improves outcome for patients with early-stage osteonecrosis of the femoral head: A comparative study. The Journal of Arthroplasty. 2015;**30**(9 Suppl):11-15

[126] Pepke W, Kasten P, Beckmann N, Janicki P, Egermann M. Core decompression and autologous bone marrow concentrate for treatment of femoral head osteonecrosis: a randomized prospective study. Orthopedic Reviews. 2016;**8**:5-9

[127] Awad ME, Hussein KA, Helwa I, Abdelsamid MF, Aguilar-Perez A, Mohsen I, et al. Meta-analysis and evidence base for the efficacy of autologous bone marrow Mesenchymal stem cells in knee cartilage repair: Methodological guidelines and quality assessment. Stem Cells International. 2019;**2019**:1-15

[128] Stein BE, Stroh DA, Schon LC. Outcomes of acute Achilles tendon rupture repair with bone marrow aspirate concentrate augmentation. International Orthopaedics. 2015;**39**(5):901-905

[129] Pascual-Garrido C, Rolón A, Makino A. Treatment of chronic patellar tendinopathy with autologous bone marrow stem cells: A 5-year-followup. Stem Cells International. 2012;**2012**:1-5

[130] Singh A, Gangwar D, Singh S. Bone marrow injection: A novel treatment for tennis elbow. Journal of Natural Science, Biology and Medicine. 2014;**5**(2):389

[131] Pettine K, Suzuki R, Sand T, Murphy M. Treatment of discogenic back pain with autologous bone marrow concentrate injection with minimum two year follow-up. International Orthopaedics. 2016;**40**(1):135-140

[132] Pettine MDK, Dordevic M, Hasz MDM. Reducing lumbar discogenic back pain and disability with intradiscal injection of bone marrow concentrate: 5-year follow-up. American Journal of Stem Cell Research. 2018;**2**(1):1-4

[133] Navani A, Manchikanti L, Albers SL, Latchaw RE, Sanapati J, Kaye AD, et al. Responsible, safe, and effective use of biologics in the management of low back pain: American Society of Interventional Pain Physicians (ASIPP) guidelines. Pain Physician. 2019;**22**:S1-S74

[134] Hart R, Komzák M, Okál F, Náhlík D, Jajtner P, Puskeiler M. Allograft alone versus allograft with bone marrow concentrate for the healing of the instrumented posterolateral lumbar fusion. The Spine Journal: The Official Journal of the North American Spine Society. 2014;**14**(7):1318-1324

[135] Yang M, Sheng L, Zhang TR, Li Q. Stem cell therapy for lower extremity diabetic ulcers: Where do we

stand? BioMed Research International. 2013;**2013**:1-8

[136] Lawall H, Bramlage P, Amann B. Stem cell and progenitor cell therapy in peripheral artery disease: A critical appraisal. Thrombosis and Haemostasis. 2010;**103**(04):696-709

[137] Balaji S, Keswani SG, Crombleholme TM. The role of mesenchymal stem cells in the regenerative wound healing phenotype. Advances in Wound Care. 2012;**1**(4):159-165

[138] Parikh PP, Liu Z-J, Velazquez OC. A molecular and clinical review of stem cell therapy in critical limb ischemia. Stem Cells International. 2017;**2017**:1-10

[139] Uccioli L, Meloni M, Izzo V, Giurato L, Merolla S, Gandini R. Critical limb ischemia: Current challenges and future prospects. Vascular Health and Risk Management. 2018;**14**:63-74

[140] Ko SH, Bandyk DF. Therapeutic angiogenesis for critical limb ischemia. Seminars in Vascular Surgery. 2014;**27**(1):23-31

Chapter 2

Adipose-Derived Stem Cells (ADSCs) and Growth Differentiation Factor 11 (GDF11): Regenerative and Antiaging Capacity for the Skin

Loubna Mazini, Luc Rochette and Gabriel Malka

Abstract

Adipose-derived stem cells (ADSCs) have proven their efficiency in wound healing and skin regeneration *in vitro* and *in vivo*. They were reported to differentiate into skin cell types and migrate to wounded sites to restore cell deficiencies and functions. Secretome of ADSCs is involved in the migration and proliferation of dermal fibroblasts (DFs) and keratinocytes where growth differentiation factor 11 (GDF11) and transforming growth factor-β (TGF-β) are expected to play the principal role. Both factors are implicated in immune responses, skin cell differentiation, proliferation and pigmentation, migration and secretion of the extracellular matrix proteins. Increasing evidence has pointed the fact that ADSCs are expected to cross-react with GDF11 to ensure DF and keratinocytes proliferation to reverse the aging process. Moreover, these factors share similar intracellular mechanisms pathways that are SMAD-dependent, and target different cellular mechanisms related to regeneration or rejuvenation. This intriguing balance between GDF11-dependent aging and TGF-β-dependent regeneration still remains unclear and might be regulated in a spatio-temporal manner. Considering the clinical relevance of the mechanisms slowing or delaying the onset of age, we aimed to clarify the involvement of cell signaling pathways related to GDF11 and TGF-β in balancing cell rejuvenation and cell regeneration. Increasing the organ lifespan and functionality might be challenging issues.

Keywords: adipose-derived stem cells, skin, aging, regeneration, rejuvenation, wound healing, GDF11, TGF-β, SMAD pathways

1. Introduction

Skin covers the human body and acts as a protective barrier against external aggressions; it consists of three component layers: epidermis, dermis, and hypodermis. Skin also has a pivotal role in thermoregulation, water retention, and cell regeneration. However, the skin remains the first exhibition of time passing characterized externally by skin winkles' manifestations, loss of integrity elasticity and functionality. These processes vary between individuals but altogether reflect cellular and molecular changes leading to progressive reduction in cell proliferation and regeneration as a result of increasing cell senescence and apoptosis [1].

A recent work has testified that adult multipotent stem cells are present in the dermal sheets and in the interfollicular dermis; they can also be derived from the pericytes [2]. They are expected to play a crucial role in regulating skin function and turnover. Furthermore, these cells were considered as mesenchymal stem cell (MSC)-like expressing the specific mesenchymal markers and differentiating into adipocyte, chondrocyte, osteoblast and myocyte [3]. These cells are identified within the subcutaneous adipose tissue as adipose-derived stem cells (ADSCs) and have been reported to differentiate into skin cells, thus ensuring skin regeneration and maintaining homeostasis [4–6]. Several studies have shown the ability of ADSCs to act through cell-cell contact, but mostly by secreting a panel of cytokines and chemokines, being involved in different biological pathways including cell proliferation, differentiation, homing and migration, senescence, and apoptosis [7–11]. These mechanisms are implicated in the whole process of skin regeneration during wound healing.

ADSC-based therapy is very promising in treating damaged tissues and in completing full-thickness skin replacement. Some clinical applications benefit from its simple and abundant collection from adipose tissue. The capacity of these cells to proliferate and self-renew *in vitro* as well as *in vitro* added to their innate differentiation has targeted more scientific advancements in the field of regenerative medicine. Their immunomodulatory effects also make them more suitable for use compared to their counterpart from bone marrow and umbilical cord blood [12]. These cells have been used for many investigations and are largely used for graft improvement in cosmetic remodeling to prevent fat necrosis [13–15]. ADSCs have presented a great ability to migrate and were recruited rapidly into wounded sites where the process of cell differentiation toward various skin cell components occurred. ADSCs have helped in cicatrization and regulating inflammation and the phases of wound healing [6]. These cells secrete growth factors in their extracellular vesicles [16–18] and produce different amounts of the extracellular matrix (ECM) proteins, thus promoting and accelerating skin regeneration in 3D raft cultures from adult expanded human skin [19, 20]. This suggested that these cells represent a rich source of factors necessary for accelerating wound healing and tissue regeneration.

Among the secreted growth factors, transforming growth factor-β (TGF-β) and growth differentiation factor 11 (GDF11) are highlighted and both are involved in biology of skin and different organs [5, 21, 22]. Both factors belong to the same superfamily of TGF-β and target similar skin cells including dermal fibroblast (DF), keratinocytes, melanocytes, and dermal microvascular endothelial cells [23–25]. Moreover, these factors activate the intracellular SMAD signaling pathways, thus targeting skin cell properties to repair wounded tissues. Consequently, TGF-β reduces wrinkles and photoaging signs [24, 26, 27]. On the other hand, GDF11 has received more attention with its ability to produce age-reversing effects [25, 28] and increase skin cell proliferation and functionality [23–25].

In the current research, many questions have been raised about the involvement of GDF11 in the inflammatory, proliferative, and remodeling phases of wound healing. Adding to the fact that TGF-β was secreted by utmost epithelial cells and participated extensively in this cascade, an interaction between GDF11 and TGF-β for sustainable skin biology and function has been suggested. Additionally, they share similar intracellular mechanisms involved in healing and aging. Cross-talking with the surrounding cells, mainly resident ADSCs, keratinocytes, DF, melanocytes, and macrophages, these factors might be activated, autoactivated, and/or mediate other cytokines and chemokines to attain and orchestrate even similar mechanism pathways but taking advantage for skin repair and cell regeneration or cell rejuvenation through resident's stem cell proliferation and differentiation.

When secreting TGF-β and GDF11, ADSCs underwent autoinduction by binding these factors to their transmembrane specific receptors ActIIBR and TGF-βR respectively and initiating the intracellular signal transduction cascade. However, circulating GDF11 has been reported to decrease with age [21, 29] and, in the same way, younger ADSCs and MSCs were found to be more proliferative, secrete more ECM proteins, and be more rejuvenating as compared to the aged ones [18]. On the other hand, positive effects on skin vasculature, skin integrity, density and strength, and wrinkles reduction have been reported when using recombinant GDF11 (rGDF11) [24] likely by cross-talk between DF, keratinocytes, ADSCs, and endothelial cells. Its beneficial involvement in skin microvasculature impaired during aging is highly expected through proliferation and differentiation of progenitor endothelial cells [30]. Other reports suggested that TGF-β was more involved in skin repair and cell regeneration during normal biological process or after injury and is considered as a key tool in the regulation of wound healing by promoting angiogenesis, cell proliferation, and migration [31]. Through its immunoregulating capacity, TFG-β and GDF11 were also specifically implicated in skin inflammatory process during wound healing and skin aging or inflamm-aging by downregulating proinflammatory cytokine genes expression [32, 33].

However, the relationships between TGF-β and GDF11 are not fully understood. With regard to their secretion levels and the skin regeneration and youth during aging, an expected ratio of TFG-β/GDF11 might be considered and regulated in a spatio-temporal manner and balance the whole cellular and molecular mechanisms associated to regeneration or rejuvenation. These regulating aspects must draw more attention as an important potential target attaining antiaging processes during wound healing.

2. Skin: anatomy and physiology

Skin thickness varies between people and with age and ranges on average from 0.05 to 2 mm. Skin is comprised of three layers: non-vascularized and stratified epidermis, underlying the dermis composed of a connective tissue and the subcutaneous adipose tissue forming the hypodermis including the adnexal structure [34]. The epidermis is preceded by an organized structure the *stratum corneum* formed by as interdigitated dead cells called corneocytes disposed as bricks between multiple lipid bilayers holding the structure defined as "brick and mortar" [35] and represent the first barrier to external factor penetration. The viable layers of the epidermis are *stratum lucidum*, *stratum granulosum*, *stratum spinosum*, and *stratum germinativum*. Keratinocytes composing these layers undergo progressive differentiation from the basal *stratum germinativum* to the outermost layer. These self-renewal and differentiation processes are important for epidermal regeneration and lead to generation of solid lipid-rich cornified layers [36]. Melanocytes are other cells present in the epidermis; they synthetize the melanin pigment being transferred to mature keratinocytes, providing principal skin protection against UV damages. Merkel cells, dendritic cells, adipocytes, and Langerhans cells are also present within the epidermis.

Fibroblasts are the principal cells constituting the dermis; they are mesenchymal and represent skin scaffolds where they support other epithelial cells and the epidermis through their elongation and shaped form, but especially through secretion of fibrous and elastic components constituting the ECM responsible for cutaneous strength and elasticity [34]. ECM is composed of fibrous proteins and a ground substance. Both these components are rearranged to provide a three-dimensional microenvironment where epithelial cells, stem cells, and the vascular network are closely related to collagen, elastin, and fibronectin fibers [37]. In human skin, collagen fibers, mostly type I, III, and V, are the dominant components in the ECM accounting for 75% of the dry skin weight and confer elasticity and strength. Type I collagen represents 80–90% of the total collagen and type III up to 8–12% while type V collagen represents the remaining minor proportion [38]. ECM not only provides a structural support for skin cells but also plays very critical role in regulating cell behavior in normal conditions and wound healing [39]. This regulation occurs through molecular signaling mediated by integrin cell surface, which orients cells toward proliferation, differentiation, migration, or apoptosis [40].

Additional skin components residing in the dermis and sometimes in the hypodermis are immune cells represented by lymphocytes, macrophages, mast and dendritic cells. Adnexal structures are located in the dermis and hypodermis and include hair follicles, blood vessels, nerves, eccrine glands, sebaceous glands, and apocrine gland.

The hypodermis layer or subcutaneous layer is composed mostly by adipose tissue containing adipocytes, stem cells (ADSCs), and blood and lymph vessels. This adipose tissue is the main actor in regulating skin homeostasis, thermoregulation, metabolism, immune responses, and immunomodulation through a wide range of cytokines and chemokines secreted. This secretory panel conditions the microenvironment of the surrounding ADSCs and consequently their secretome to modulate skin cell proliferation, differentiation, migration, melanin production, and to induce skin rejuvenation [41–43].

3. Skin aging

3.1 Mechanisms of skin aging

Skin aging dependent on age or photoaging represents actually a real challenge of the new ADSCs advancements. The apparent skin physiology and morphology represent the first signal of cell aging. Skin aging is represented by epidermal atrophy, wrinkles appearance, reduction of dermal thickness, and ECM degradation; adnexal structures also decrease in their number and function. Decrease in the number of epithelial cells including DF, melanocytes, and Langerhans cells was reported as well. Their replicative ability decreases with age, leading to senescent and non-dividing cells.

The thickness of subcutaneous adipose tissue is also reduced, showing a decrease in mitotic activity and self-renewal of ADSCs and increase in senescence of the surrounding cells. ADSCs might behave differently according to the context of stimulation, but the mainly important factors that are relayed to cell proliferation, proinflammation, and angiogenesis altogether are involved in cell regeneration.

3.2 Physiological markers of skin aging

We believe now that aging is associated to many intrinsic signaling pathway related to epigenetic factors, some genetic predispositions, and extrinsic factors such as ultraviolet radiations, air and water pollution, resulting in the impairment of skin integrity and youth. One could consider that UV/infrared (IR) irradiations might lead to more cell damage than intrinsic factors. Indeed, following IR irradiation, skin cells present different DNA damages. Also, wrinkles, elasticity loss, pigmentation dysfunction, or hyperkeratosis are the most common symptoms reflecting the visual extent of aging as a result of the progressive atrophy of the dermis. These manifestations rely on the impairment of cell senescence, a multifactorial event leading to skin integrity loss. Collagen production decreases and its degradation increases, leading to a quantitative and structural change in collagen fibers, which impact the dermis structure [44–46].

In humans, GDF11 is connected to age-related diseases and its serum level is associated with the physiology of aging [47, 48]. Its circulating level has been associated with aging in many human organs [23, 49, 50]. This factor was found to be able to antagonize aging specifically [29] and its remarkable action against myocardial hypertrophy and inflammation has been largely reported [28, 51, 52].

During skin aging, keratinocytes, DF and although endothelial cells secrete ubiquitous endopeptidases able to degrade the ECM proteins and called matrix metalloproteinase (MMP). Degradation of collagen fibers occurs with the major protease present in human skin MMP-1 that degrades type I and III collagen, followed by MMP-3 and MMP-9 [53]. The specific tissue inhibitors of metalloproteinases (TIMPs) regulate MMP processes where their increase in levels during aging was not concomitant with that of TIMPs leading to intrinsic collagen deficiency and accelerated skin aging. Moreover, Patel et al. have suggested that the ratio of MMP/TIMPs could be considered as a biomarker of wound healing and aging [54]. In photoaging, elastic fiber disorganization and degradation were observed, mainly due to activation of MMP-2, MMP-3, MMP-9, MMP-12, and MMP-13 [45, 55, 56]. UVA-treated fibroblasts presented a typical senescence phenotype including upregulation of α-SMA, MMP-1, and MMP-2 expression [25].

Behind the increase in MMP levels, another component generated in skin cells is represented by reactive oxygen species (ROS). When activating the mitogen-activated protein kinase (MAPK) family, transcriptional factors such as activator protein 1 (AP-1) and nuclear factor-kB (NF-kB) induce upregulation of MMP in DF and keratinocytes [57–60]. In addition, when cells aged, dysfunctions of mitochondrial electron transport chains and a decrease in mitochondrial activity were reported leading to higher production of ROS [61, 62]. Accumulation of ROS induced oxidative damages of structural proteins and lipoproteins, thus favoring cell senescence. On the other hand, this senescence might also be induced by the decline in replicative capacity due to DNA damage, including DNA methylation, histone deacetylation, or to chromatine architecture change and to gene expression which compromise the intended cellular function. The increase in mitochondrial ROS generation was also correlated to the decrease in DF size and spreading observed during progressive ECM degradation and impaired DF attachment due probably to the involvement of MMP production [57, 63, 64].

ROS also regulated different biological mechanisms including generation of inflammatory responses. Indeed, aging is associated to an increased secretion of proinflammatory proteins such as interleukin-6 (IL-6) and matrix metalloproteinase (MMP)-9, leading to immune changes. Prolonged release of ROS in skin might amplify the inflammatory injury and promote chronic inflammation [65].

Some transcription factors such as P63 (P53 related protein) and $P16^{INK4a}$ are reported as indicators of keratinocytes senescence. Indeed, expression of $P16^{INK4a}$ positive cells increased with chronological aging in human dermis and epidermis while P63 expression was reduced [66, 67].

4. Role of ADSCs in skin regeneration

During normal development, skin regeneration is performed by the resident ADSCs providing for cellular turnover during skin homeostasis and repair after injury [41]. The basal layer is the skin location where these active multipotent stem cells are responsible for recruiting and sending mature differentiated cells (keratinocytes) to the outer layer of epidermis. Through a hierarchic gradient, these stem cells induced the regeneration of epidermis layer by ensuring self-renewal and a continuous production of transient amplifying cells [68]. Epidermal cells including ADSCs and DF closely interact to maintain local microenvironment propitious for cell turnover, leading to skin regeneration. Adding to their tendency to differentiate into keratinocytes, DF, and probably melanocytes, cross-talk of ADSCs and these cells is a part of normal skin function where ECM secretion leads to a physical environment critical for the maintenance of the stem cell niche [69].

Another proof of the interactions between fibroblasts and ADSCs has been provided by Hu et al. where skin fibroblasts cell line HS27 was found to activate ADSCs to differentiate into fibroblast-like cells highly expressing vimentin, HSP47, and desmin mRNA level [70]. The interactions of microvascular endothelial cells and ADSCs are also of great interest in skin cell regeneration and proliferation by providing IL-6, IL-8, monocyte chemoattractant protein-1 (MCP-1) and VEGF, leading to inflammation and angiogenesis regulation [71, 72]. In normal conditions, ADSCs are continuously activated by human serum and platelets to induce their proliferation and differentiation. While in wounded tissues, platelets induced stem cells to initiate the inflammatory phase by secreting platelet-derived growth factor (PDGF), IL-6 and IL-8, which lead to migration of macrophages and neutrophils to the wounded site [73], and TGF-β inducing induction of monocytes to macrophages (**Figure 1**).

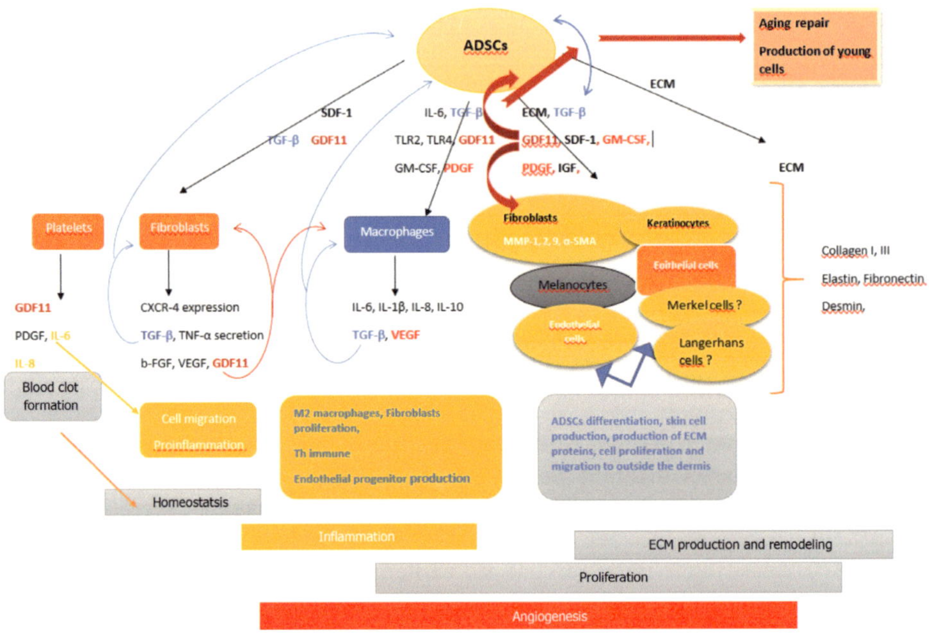

Figure 1.
Implication of adipose-derived stem cells in the different phases associated to wound healing and in the rejuvenation process. ADSCs act on fibroblasts, macrophages, and skin cells through their secreted growth factors. GDF11 and TGF-β are present in all the phases, amplify fibroblast, macrophage, and ADSC secretion, leading to immune response, cell proliferation, and angiogenesis. However, their interactions are more relevant during proliferation phases where GDF11 might induce TFG-β induction in a spatio-temporal manner in addition to boosting fibroblast proliferation, resulting in the production of skin cell presenting young profile. GDF11: growth differentiation factor, TGF-β: transforming growth factor, ECM: extracellular matrix, PDGF: platelets-derived growth factor, Il-1,6,8,10: interleukin-1, TNF-α: tumor necrosis factor-α, b-FGF: basic-fibroblast growth factor, VEGF: vascular endothelial growth factor, CXCR-4: C motif chemokine receptor 4, SDF-1: stromal derived factor-1, TLR2, 4: toll-like receptor2,4, GM-CSF: granulocyte monocyte-colony stimulating factor, IGF: insulin growth factor, MMP-1,-2, -9: matrix metalloproteinase-1, -2, -9, α-SMA: α-smooth muscle actin.

Similar to platelets, ADSCs additionally secrete prostaglandin E2 (PGE2), TNF-α, and GDF11, thus potentiating proinflammatory responses and later anti-inflammatory cytokine secretion by polarizing macrophages from M1 to M2.

In addition to TGF-β and GDF11, ADSCs secrete other growth factors such as basic-fibroblast Growth Factor (b-FGF), stromal-derived factor-1 (SDF-1), insulin-like growth factor (IGF), hepatocyte growth factor (HGF), and wingless 10b (Wnt10b), which are involved in the mechanisms regulating skin cell regeneration and repair [10, 23, 74]. The factors VEGF, PDGF, TGF-β, b-FGF, and HGF induce the formation of new blood vessels during the proliferative phase, probably through their differentiation into endothelial progenitor cells [10, 75]. The secreted GM-CSF can take part in this activation by inducing differentiation into committed monocytes potentially activated to macrophages and endothelial cells. In chronic radiation wounds, the use of ADSCs promoted new blood vessels damaged by the irradiation and increased the capillary density. These cells were found to act through stimulation of fibroblast proliferation and increase in VEGF secretion level [76].

However, endothelial cells and macrophages migration have been possible once after macrophages leaded to secretion of the ECM proteins especially collagen I and III, elastin and fibronectin and to activation of DF to proliferate and migrate. DF also secretes VEGF, TGF-β, and b-FGF, leading to angiogenesis [75, 77]. ADSCs are expected to participate actively in ECM production, whereby its abundant accumulation would facilitate cell migration and angiogenesis by autoinduction and amplification of the growth factor secretion implied. When miming injured conditions *in vitro*, ADSCs were indeed demonstrated to accelerate neovascularization through the expression of hypoxia-inducible factor-1α [78] by regulating VEGF gene expression in endothelial cells [79]. These observations were confirmed *in vitro* in addition to an activation of stem cell proliferation and to keratinocytes chemoattraction and migration [80] likely facilitated by MMPs [81].

Migration of ADSCs to the injured site is of pivotal interest; their immune profile and their potential shift toward a more anti-inflammatory phenotype is required for the proliferation and remodeling phases of healing [82–84]. The cytokine profile of T, B, and dendritic cells was influenced by ADSCs, which lead to the interruption of the inflammatory phase and starting the proliferation and remodeling phases in chronic wounds [6, 85, 86]. The potential involvement of GDF11 in disrupting the proinflammatory status toward the anti-inflammatory one is likely due to its highly stimulation of DF and ADSCs and also by amplifying the action of TGF-β on ADSCs proliferation and secretome. This epigenetic modification and regulation of ADSCs' microenvironment might be crucial in restoring cellular age defects and/or increasing cells' ability to differentiate and migrate. The impact of changing microenvironment on induction of cell proliferation, differentiation, and migration has already been reported [41–43].

The collagen production amplified by cross-talk between ADSCs, DF, and TGF-β would facilitate the remodeling phase through inhibiting ECM degradation by increasing TIMPs' secretion and their binding to MMPs [87]. Xiao et al. have reported that adipose tissue secretome increased N-cadherin and CD44 adhesion molecules involved in fibroblasts' motility during wound healing and stimulation of fibronectin expression during ECM remodeling [88]. Combination of activin B and ADSCs led to rapid wound closure and to accelerated epithelialization through promoting keratinocytes and fibroblasts proliferation [5]. The integrin αβ6 exclusively expressed by epithelial cells was associated to the regeneration of basement membrane zone during wound repair [89].

Figure 1 summarizes ADSCs' mechanisms involved in tissue repair.

5. ADSCs' interactions with TFG-β and GDF11 for skin regeneration

Increasing evidence has implicated ADSCs in maintaining skin homeostasis at a cellular level through cell differentiation and at the paracrine level. The exosomes they secrete respond to the hemostasis of skin microenvironment by releasing the growth factors promoting neo-angiogenesis, cell differentiation, cell proliferation, and migration [11, 16, 90–92].

5.1 Proliferation and differentiation of ADSCs into skin cells

Through their secreting growth factors, ADSCs impacted cell proliferation, migration, and senescence, which are the physiological parameters associated with wound injury and aging. During wound healing, ADSCs and DF have been reported to optimize and address their local environment, the secreted ECM proteins have been reported to modulate the activity of keratinocytes and DF through mediating secretion of growth factors such as TGF-β to activate the healing process [41–43, 69]. TGF-β plays a critical role in ECM protein production and especially collagen synthesis and degradation via the SMAD pathway [44]. Sasaki et al. were the first to identify the implication of MSCs in skin regeneration by their ability to differentiate and to repopulate damaged tissues [93]. Also, green fluorescent protein (GFP)-positive bone marrow MSCs were able to differentiate into keratinocytes, endothelial cells, and pericytes presenting altogether specific cell line markers [42].

Nevertheless, other factors are secreted by ADSCs or other epithelial cells that were recently identified to pave the way to the ones reported above or even have a place of honor in favoring skin regeneration or rejuvenation. In regard to this fact, the first on the list might be the GDF11, another member of the TGF-β family recently involved in the structural and functional amelioration of skin cell and supporting skin stem cell proliferation and differentiation [23, 24].

GDF11, also known as bone morphogenetic protein-11 (BMP-11), is a disulfide-linked dimer existing in a proactive form maturing after cleavage by furin-like proteases with 407 amino acids. This factor is expressed in embryonic tissues while mRNA and protein levels were differently appreciated with higher protein levels in soft tissue, cerebral cortex, adrenal gland, testis, and hippocampus [5]. Many physiological and pathophysiological functions are attributed to this factor, including cell embryonic development, erythropoiesis, proliferation and differentiation, cardiovascular diseases, diabetes mellitus, and age-related diseases [5, 94].

However, the mostly important fact reported is that secreting GDF11 by ADSC originates the mechanisms related to cell differentiation and proliferation and cell migration even by upregulating genes involved in skin barrier function, in cellular proliferation, to epidermal turnover and differentiation and via modulating the TGF-β/SMAD pathway. Genes related to ECM production were also found upregulated after Smad2 and Smad3 activation, in parallel to decrease in IL-1β proinflammatory cytokine-related gene [24]. Indeed, DF produced TGF-β and GDF11 [95, 96] in addition to laminin, collagen, elastin, and fibronectin to ensure mechanical stability of the dermis and participated to epidermis cell functions including those of keratinocytes and melanocytes. ADSCs were also reported to secrete ECM proteins participating in this activation loop.

Additionally, ADSCs might be automodulated by the secreted GDF11. On the other hand, GDF11 increased MMP-9 gene expression, which is known to interact with TGF-β to help wound closure and facilitate wound healing. However, high production of this protein is expected to improve matrix remodeling after injury rather than its degradation [97].

5.2 Skin cell migration

Subcutaneous MSCs mainly identified as ADSCs were considered as the principal actor in the process of skin cell migration [93] but their presence within skin layers has not been established yet. Additionally, adipose tissue extract containing evidently ADSC's secretome was able to significantly stimulate DF migration [25].

By expressing the chemokine receptor CCR7, which is the specific receptor of SLC/CCL21 involved in cell migration, MSCs accelerated their recruitment and migrated to the injured site, thus stimulating wound repair by giving rise to differentiated skin cells *in vivo*.

TGF-β is secreted by DF, macrophages, and ADSCs and consequently amplifies angiogenesis and migration of ADSCs, keratinocytes, and DF by stimulating the SMAD2/3 pathway and increasing the expression of CXCR-4 receptor of SDF-1. This migration has been confirmed *in vitro* while ADSCs were recruited into damaged sites by SDF-1 [98], using the SDF-1/CXCR-4 axis and the intracellular Jak/AKt regulation pathway [99]. GDF11 also stimulated DF and keratinocytes to migrate into wounded sites [23]. By activating the same SMAD2/3/pathway, GDF11 and TGF-β stimulate skin endothelial cells to migrate, thus improving angiogenesis. This suggested that GDF11 activates the identical pathway in other skin cells such as DF and keratinocytes to improve cell migration and wound repair [24].

Other mechanisms leading to ADSC migration were reported after their activation by activin B, JRK, and ERK signaling appeared to be responsible for actin stress fiber formation involved in cell migration [5]. Interestingly, activin B was found to promote ADSC migration by enhancing α-SMA expression and stress fiber formation.

5.3 Melanocytes regulation

ADSCs also interplay with the activation loop of melanocytes by modulating enzyme-producing melanin activity. ADSCs by increasing their TGF-β secretion induced melanocytes to downregulate the expression of melanogenic enzymes and prevent site-specific pigmentation in reconstructed skin grafts. These interactions might be of interest in clinical applications by modulating melanin synthesis and impacting whitening of the skin through TGF-β [100]. DF increased TGF-β secretion, thus maintaining melanocytes in an immature state, and acted on melanocytes to modulate melanin-producing enzymes and thus skin pigmentation [101], suggesting that dermal composition in cells might determine the production of mature melanocytes and hence melanin transfer to keratinocytes. However, a recent study has shown that rGDF11 significantly reduced melanin production in melanocytes and 3D skin equivalents [24]. On the other hand, during aging, ROS accumulation by cell proliferation was reported as the initiator of the occurrence of vitiligo and its progression [102].

These reports might increase our thought on a potential ratio of GDF11 and TGF-β in different skin type and color. This ratio could result on a balance between skin pigmentation and skin yought and lead to a sustainable skin biology and function through regulation of the mechanisms related to skin cell proliferation and rejuvenation. If this is the case, one should conclude that white skins should present higher amounts of GDF11 and youthful aspects and present less symptoms of cell apoptosis and senescence during cell life. These observations must draw more attention in the future to better understand the paradigms triggering the mechanisms related to skin aging and pigmentation.

6. TGF-β and GDF11 impacts on immunoregulatory effects of ADSC in skin

Evidence of involvement of ADSCs in immunomodulation of tissues and their presence within the epidermal layer have suggested that these cells might play a crucial role in skin immunological functions in physiologic and injured skin. Accumulation of senescent cells is related to the production of proinflammatory factors such as IL-6, IL-8, and TNF-α; we can postulate that the associated chronic inflammation is a promoting age-associated disease due to tissue aging. This skin inflamm-aging was also supported by highly secreted proinflammatory cytokine IL-1 β [32, 33]. Microvascular endothelial cells also interact with ADSCs to increase secretion of IL-6, IL-8, and MCP-1 to modulate skin inflammation [72].

TFG-β, secreted by ADSCs and other epithelial cells, is involved in the inflammatory, proliferative, and remodeling phases of wound healing. This factor activates M2 macrophages and secretion of ECM proteins involved in skin structure repair, in angiogenesis, in DF proliferation and cell migration, and re-epithelialization.

The integrin αβ6 secreted by epithelial cells was reported to activate TGF-β modulation and thus the innate immune surveillance in skin [89]. Recently, the collagen triple helix repeat containing one protein was reported to contribute to healing process via increasing M2 macrophages recruitment and TGF-β expression level [103].

In the same way, IL-6, the major proinflammatory component of ADSC's secretome, was reported to initiate the inflammatory phase in injured tissues. Autoactivated ADSCs amplify their secretion and stimulate the secretion of TNF-α, TLR2, TLR4, IL-10, b-FGF, VEGF, TGF-β, and GDF11. These secretions would take place to short and shift the ADSCs profile to an anti-inflammatory profile and enhance angiogenesis, cell migration, and proliferation (**Figure 2**). Like TGF-β,

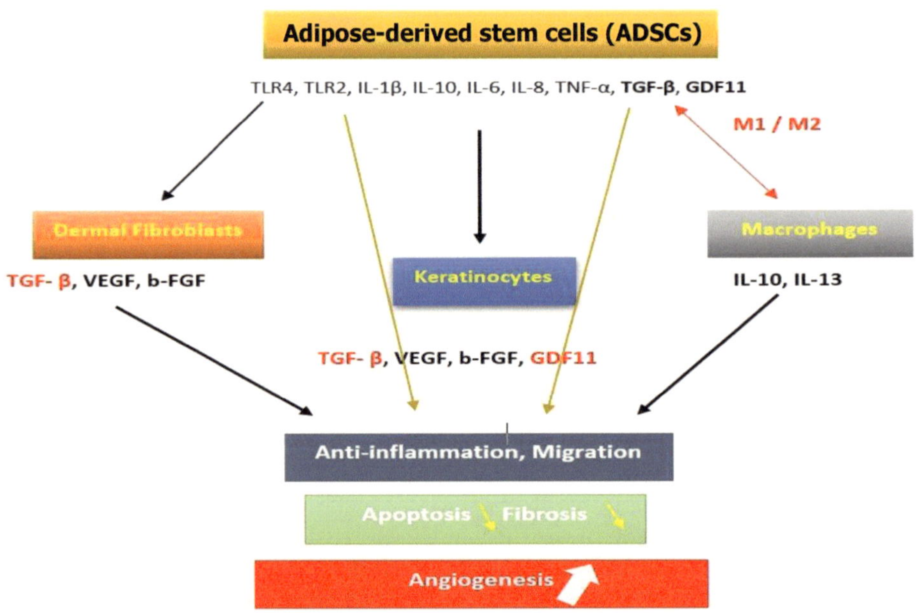

Figure 2.
Immunomodulatory effects of ADSCs. Through their secretome, these cells change the macrophages' polarization and acquire an anti-inflammatory profile to enhance skin cell proliferation and migration and accelerate angiogenesis.

GDF11 was found to be associated to the skin inflammatory status in both physiological process and injury and participate in the regulation of the immune response.

To determine the effect of GDF11 on skin inflammation, a recent work of Wang et al. has shown that skin treatment with rGDF11 decreased the secretion of inflammatory cytokines by immune cells *in vitro* and *in vivo* in mice models of psoriasis-associated inflammation, an extended infiltration of immune cells sustaining skin inflammation. Suppression of the severity of this inflammation by GDF11 was achieved by reducing macrophages infiltration to the skin and inhibiting the NF-kB signaling pathway [51]. Moreover, macrophages activation has been reported in skin autoimmune inflammatory diseases [104]. Other evidences argued on the protective effect of GDF11 from inflammatory reaction by inhibiting inflammatory responses in RAW264.7 macrophages [105], probably by inhibiting TNF-α release [106]. Additionally, TNF-α was activated by NF-kB signaling pathway during inflammation reaction, being suppressed by GDF11 in atherosclerosis. By reducing the NF-kB pathway, GDF11 also protected against apoptosis [105]. This suggested that the anti-inflammatory effect of GDF11 could open the way to potential new strategies for treating skin inflammations.

7. Antiaging mechanisms of ADSC within TFG-β and GDF11

7.1 Cellular implication

The mechanisms inducing tissue degeneration and cell aging remain multifactorial and still unclear. Senescent ADSCs were likely found to be impacted in their ability to sustain tissue hemostasis and hence resulted in loss of tissue and organ integrity. Even these cells display a rich secretory profile; their ability to secrete ECM proteins, cytokines, and chemokines was largely impaired *in vitro* during culture expansion [107].

A recent clinical study has demonstrated that secretome of adipose tissue lipoaspirate extracellular fraction stimulates epidermal and dermal cell proliferation in a dose-dependent manner. This secretome has also the ability to delay apoptosis, enhance fibroblasts proliferation and migration, and reverse specifically the aging process and the associated skin symptoms [25, 28]. Exposure of fibroblasts to UVA was followed by preventing the upregulation of MMP1, MMP2, and α-SMA expression as well as lower elastin and collagen production associated to the senescence-like phenotype [25]. Indeed, ADSCs have proven their superiority in improving and increasing dermal thickness and reducing wrinkles more likely by inducing paracrine DF and angiogenesis [17, 18, 108]. Administrated intradermally to an aged skin, skin texture and wrinkles as well as dermal thickness were found improved 8 weeks after treatment [74]. The extracellular vesicles released in ADSCs' secretome or conditioned media enable the targeted cells to increase the production and deposition of ECM proteins including collagen and elastin [11, 16, 90, 109, 110]. Among these autocrine/paracrine factors, TGF-β and GDF11 appeared to be strongly associated (**Figure 1**).

Indeed, ADSCs-conditioned media *in vitro* and *in vivo* have proven their efficiency in stimulating rejuvenation of human skin by improving skin elasticity and reducing wrinkles in a GDF11-dependent manner [111–113]. Their extract acted in a similar manner by activating DF and keratinocytes to proliferate and migrate into damaged sites [114]. An anti-wrinkle effect and dermal density increase were shown after *in vivo* treatment [23]. Moreover, the young cells secreting more GDF11 supported higher proliferation rate of keratinocyte stem cells than those from aged donors [115]. In the same manner, using platelets-rich plasma (PRP) for anti-wrinkle and anti-aging skin aspects appeared legitime related to its higher quantities of GDF11 [116]. Interestingly, GDF11 expression and activity were reduced in adult DF compared to the neonatal ones [95].

Fibroblasts were also recognized to play a crucial role in skin regeneration through GDF11 secretion in both neonatal and adult cells [95]. MSCs derived from placenta and umbilical cord blood promote fibroblasts plasticity [117] probably through GDF11 release, thus stimulating the rejuvenation of human skin [118]. These authors have effectively demonstrated that GDF11 activated fibroblasts to increase ECM proteins' production and especially collagen I and III and fibronectin [23]. Also, MSCs have proven their proliferative superiority in young donors rather than the elderly [18].

In an animal model, transplanted autologous ADSCs improved skin-graft survival through secreting factors presenting anti-apoptotic activity [119]. In addition to ADSC, DF also appeared attractive in terms of protein secretion [109]. ADSC-conditioned media were anti-apoptotic and ensured skin tissue regeneration [119]; their protective and antiaging properties have been demonstrated on DF by preventing their oxidative stress and increasing their superoxide dismutase and glutathione peroxidase activities [120]. These cells act through their different and directed secretome to improve and induce tissue repair, consolidating their place as better candidate for regenerative medicine and opening recently the way for a new cell-free therapy [109, 121].

Moreover, by increasing collagenase matrix metalloproteinase-9 (MMP-9) secretion, rGDF11 participated in matrix remodeling maybe through interaction of MMP-9 with TGF-β1 to facilitate skin wound closure [97, 122]. These cell interactions reveal the role of the TFG-β and GDF11 mechanisms used by ADSCs to interfere with the aging process [24, 95, 101].

7.2 Intracellular mechanisms pathway balancing between TGF-β and GDF11 in skin aging

Aging of ADSCs and DF was associated to upregulation of apoptotic genes and, consequently, the number of senescent cells increased [123]. However, recent studies have demonstrated that this senescence can be induced by TGF-β/SMAD as a normal developmental process [124]. Also, in aged skin, accumulation of senescent cells and ROS likely impaired TGF-B pathway at least in DF. The mechanisms' pathways SMAD and Sirtuins are the mostly reported pathways whereby TGF-β and GDF11 acted.

The sirtuins are a family engaged in metabolism regulation and in aging-associated diseases, in addition to the mechanistic target of rapamycin (mTOR) signaling [16, 62, 125]. SIRT1 upregulation was reported to delay fibroblast's senescence and its expression is significantly reduced in aged skin [126]. Additionally, SIRT1, SIRT3, SIRT5, SIRT2, SIRT6, and SIRT7 are involved in the regulation of oxidative stress and ROS production [127, 128]. Moreover, SIRT6 is implicated in the relation of DNA repair proteins to chromatin [129].

In wound healing, phosphorylation of TGF-β/Smad2/3 intracellular pathways was increased and resulted in protein transfer to skin cell [16, 130, 131], in DF proliferation and ADSCs differentiation into fibroblasts [70], and in improvement of angiogenesis [24]. Interestingly, aging and cell differentiation have been reversed by inhibiting this pathway [132]. Indeed, activation of SMAD2/3-dependent-TGF-β signaling inhibits adipogenic and osteogenic MSCs' differentiation *in vitro* and *in vivo* [133, 134].

DOI: http://dx.doi.org/10.5772/intechopen.91233

ADSCs self-renew is regulated by AKT signaling through targeting PDGFA and activating the PI3K/AKT2 axis is required for ADSCs proliferation and maintenance in the dermis [135]. Hypoxic conditions might play a pivotal role in wound repair, and the same pathway has been found leading to the activation of PI3K/AKt signaling [130]. In response to wound, ERK, AKt, and STAT-3 mechanisms pathways were activated and associated to stem cell proliferation and keratinocyte migration [80]. Interestingly, wound healing was specifically associated to microRNA and protein transfer to skin cells through the TGF-β/SMAD2 pathway, TGF-β being identified as a "mediator" [16, 132, 136].

TGF-β signaling pathway was recently reported as the main regulator of pluripotency [137]. Although epigenetically lacking myostatin is a highly homologous factor of GDF11, muscle multipotent stem cells can be reprogrammed to became pluripotent cells as embryonic cell-like. MicroRNA participates in this regulation probably by inhibiting TGF-β/Smad2 [132]. Epithelial differentiation was achieved by ADSCs through secreting Wnt10b and Wnt3a, a modulator of the Wnt/β-catenin implicated in replicative senescence regulation, suggesting that the regenerating and rejuvenating effect of GDF11 might also act via Wnt/β-catenin activation [138]. However, further investigations should be conducted to increase the knowledge on the intracellular mechanism used by the Wnt/β-catenin to delay the senescence of ADSCs and other targeted cells.

GDF11 is likely expected to act on other epidermal cells including DF, keratinocytes, and melanocytes by regulating the genetic expressions of the different proteins involved in the antiaging process. Recombinant GDF11 was likely reported to reinforce human skin by highly increasing ECM genes expression related to ECM production such as COL1A1, COL6A6, CL14A1, ELN, TGFBR3, and HAS1. Skin barrier function was likely improved by enhancing expression of ALOX12, ALOX12B, ALOXE3, DSG1, and DSP genes. Genes related to epidermal cell proliferation and differentiation were also upregulated in human skin through the Smad2/3mechanisms pathways [24].

Recently, fibroblast growth factors (FGFs) have been proposed as a therapeutic option to avoid skin aging aspects and to counter the cellular responses related to aging [139, 140]. Binding to tyrosine kinase receptors, they activate the autophosphorylation of Raf-1 belonging to the family of mitogen-activated protein kinase, kinase, kinase (MAPKKK), followed by that of MAPKK, which phosphorylates ERK (belonging to MAPK). Phosphorylation of these cyclin-dependent kinases in cell nucleus is involved in controlling cell division.

These FGFs are derived from fibroblasts and are decreased during their proliferative and metabolic activities, thus reducing ECM proteins' production. The decrease in FGF production also converge on the reduced amounts of collagen, decrease of dermal and epidermal integrity and elasticity and strength as signs of aging [141]. In addition to FGF secretion, fibroblasts are also targeted by TFG-β and GDF11 to activate the SMAD pathway leading them to have a pivotal role in skin regeneration. This suggests that FGF was expected to act independently but simultaneously to TGF-β and GDF11 to improve skin structure and aging aspects. Having a high mitogenic activity and high stability, rFGF-1 has been reported to strongly activate fibroblasts and keratinocytes proliferation with a potential use in angiogenesis, wound healing, and skin antiaging [142, 143]. In the same way, FGF-2 or b-FGF and keratinocyte growth factor (KGF) reduced wrinkles and increased proliferation of fibroblasts and keratinocytes modulating normal process of angiogenesis, tissue repair, and wound healing as well as significantly improving the antiaging process [27, 144, 145].

8. The spatio-temporal role of the TFG-β pathway in relationship with GDF11 in skin aging

When stimulating ADSCs through binding to their specific receptor membrane, activin type IIB (ActIIBR), GDF11 activates the SMAD2/3 pathways. Similar mechanism might be achieved on ADSCs by TGF-β, suggesting that interference with TGF-β and GDF11 mechanisms might be the key regulator of healing and aging. The same activated SMAD mechanisms pathway did not achieve similar biological activity and targeted probably different intracellular and intranuclear effectors. These considerations might suggest that even different specific receptors are involved in the extracellular interactions of these factors, a competitive attractivity might be observed between their intracellular effectors, which are the SMAD 2/3 proteins. When the factors compete for these proteins, one can speculate that the favored pathway would be associated either to the amount of the activated receptor (TGF-β or GDF11) or to the sensibility of these receptors to their respective ligands.

Another point of view that could be important to mention is the variation in secretion level of these factors during aging. At this fact, serum level of GDF11 has been reported to decrease during age while TGF-β variation was not really investigated. The antiaging pathway GDF11-dependent could be replaced progressively during aging by the TGF-β regenerating one. This might favor tissue regeneration and repair rather than rejuvenation, leading to the appearance of the symptoms of age.

Thus complicating the dilemma between rejuvenation and regeneration. Secretome composition of ADSCs might be impacted by the aging process or the different epigenetic factors.

9. Conclusion

In wound defects, ADSCs presented a great ability in migration and were recruited rapidly into wounded sites where the process of cell differentiation toward various skin cell components occurred. However, ADSCs participate more likely in all the phases of wound healing through autocrine and paracrine pathways [6]. Otherwise, during aging, senescent cells increase and the paracrine senescent secretome of ADSCs can trigger and reinforce senescence within their microenvironment [124]. This paracrine effect can be transmitted by ligands of TGF-β by mediating changes in the transcriptional program through SMAD family members [146].

Another surprising capacity of these cells is that secretome derived from younger cells is more suitable to increase proliferation than that derived from older cell [18], suggesting that younger cells have the potential to secrete a youth growth factor identified as GDF11, able to quantitatively increase cell proliferation at the younger stage. Targeted cells are the other crucial parameters leading to this increase; younger cells presented less senescence characteristics including DNA damage and ROS accumulation, thus, inducing cell rejuvenation. This process might be used to directly induce secretome of these cells toward tissue regeneration or rejuvenation.

We cannot exclude that MSCs and ADSCs secreted other cytokines than GDF11 and TGF-β, such as PDGF, IL-1, bone morphogenic protein (BMP)6, BMP9, and exerted autocrine and paracrine effects on DF and keratinocytes, promoting cell differentiation, proliferation, and migration. Nevertheless, the antiaging paracrine effect seemed to be induced, perhaps not exclusively but at least to a significant degree, by a combinatorial effect of both GDF11 and TGF-β. It is probable that both signals vary with age and that the strength of each of them is reciprocal to the sites of secreted signals and to the length of the exposure to the signal. Based on these considerations, further investigations on TGF-β and GDF11 molecular mechanisms' implication on skin rejuvenation are needed to increase our knowledge and draw conclusions on the regulation of aging process. Exciting therapeutic approaches might arise from the implication of GDF11 as an antiaging mechanism to increase the lifespan and the long-lasting functionality of different organs.

Acknowledgements

The authors wish to thank the University of Mohammed VI Polytechnic for funding this work.

Conflict of interest

The authors declare no conflict of interest.

List of abbreviations

ADSCs	adipose-derived stem cells
GDF11	growth differentiation factor
TGF-β	transforming growth factor
ECM	extracellular matrix
DF	dermal fibroblasts
ROS	reactive oxygen species
MSCs	mesenchymal stem cells
MMP1, 2, 9	matrix metalloproteinase1, 2, 9
IL-1, −6, −8, −10	interleukin-1, −6, −8, −10
TNF-α	tumor necrosis factor-α
VEGF	vascular endothelial growth factor
PDGF	platelets derived growth factor
α-SMA	α-smooth muscle actin
MCP-1	monocyte chemoattractant protein-1

Author details

Loubna Mazini[1*], Luc Rochette[2] and Gabriel Malka[1]

1 Laboratoire Cellules Souches et Ingénierie Tissulaire, Centre Interface Applications Médicales (CIAM), Mohammed VI Polytechnic University, Ben Guérir, Morocco

2 Equipe d'Accueil (EA 7460): Physiopathologie et Epidémiologie Cérébro-Cardiovasculaires (PEC2), Faculté des Sciences de Santé, Université de Bourgogne Franche Comté, Dijon, France

*Address all correspondence to: loubna.mazini@um6p.ma

References

[1] DiLoreto R, Murphy CT. The cell biology of aging. Molecular Biology of the Cell. 2015;**26**:4524-4531

[2] Hu MS, Borrelli MR, Lorenz HP, Longaker MT, Wan DC. Mesenchymal stromal cells and cutaneous wound healing: A comprehensive review of the background, role, and therapeutic potential. Stem Cells International. 2018;**2018**:6901983

[3] Rodriguez A-M, Elabd C, Amri E-Z, Ailhaud G, Dani C. The human adipose tissue is a source of multipotent stem cells. Biochimie. 2005;**87**:125-128

[4] Marfia G, Navone SE, Di Vito C, Ughi N, Tabano S, Miozzo M, et al. Mesenchymal stem cells: Potential for therapy and treatment of chronic non-healing skin wounds. Organogenesis. 2015;**11**:183-206

[5] Zhang Y, Wei Y, Liu D, Liu F, Li X, Pan L, et al. Role of growth differentiation factor 11 in development, physiology and disease. Oncotarget. 2017;**8**:81604-81616

[6] Hyldig K, Riis S, Pennisi CP, Zachar V, Fink T. Implications of extracellular matrix production by adipose tissue-derived stem cells for development of wound healing therapies. International Journal of Molecular Sciences. 31 May 2017;**18**(6)

[7] Balaji S, Keswani SG, Crombleholme TM. The role of mesenchymal stem cells in the regenerative wound healing phenotype. Advances in Wound Care (New Rochelle). 2012;**1**:159-165

[8] Amable PR, Teixeira MVT, Carias RBV, Granjeiro JM, Borojevic R. Protein synthesis and secretion in human mesenchymal cells derived from bone marrow, adipose tissue and Wharton's jelly. Stem Cell Research & Therapy. 2014;**5**:53

[9] Elman JS, Li M, Wang F, Gimble JM, Parekkadan B. A comparison of adipose and bone marrow-derived mesenchymal stromal cell secreted factors in the treatment of systemic inflammation. Journal of Inflammation (Lond). 2014;**11**:1

[10] Kilroy GE, Foster SJ, Wu X, Ruiz J, Sherwood S, Heifetz A, et al. Cytokine profile of human adipose-derived stem cells: Expression of angiogenic, hematopoietic, and pro-inflammatory factors. Journal of Cellular Physiology. 2007;**212**:702-709

[11] Choi EW, Seo MK, Woo EY, Kim SH, Park EJ, Kim S. Exosomes from human adipose-derived stem cells promote proliferation and migration of skin fibroblasts. Experimental Dermatology. 2018;**27**:1170-1172

[12] Gonzalez-Rey E, Anderson P, González MA, Rico L, Büscher D, Delgado M. Human adult stem cells derived from adipose tissue protect against experimental colitis and sepsis. Gut. 2009;**58**:929-939

[13] Koh KS, Oh TS, Kim H, Chung IW, Lee KW, Lee HB, et al. Clinical application of human adipose tissue-derived mesenchymal stem cells in progressive hemifacial atrophy (Parry-Romberg disease) with microfat grafting techniques using 3-dimensional computed tomography and 3-dimensional camera. Annals of Plastic Surgery. 2012;**69**:331-337

[14] Bae YC, Song JS, Bae SH, Kim JH. Effects of human adipose-derived stem cells and stromal vascular fraction on cryopreserved fat transfer. Dermatologic Surgery. 2015;**41**:605-614

[15] Eto H, Kato H, Suga H, Aoi N, Doi K, Kuno S, et al. The fate of adipocytes after nonvascularized fat grafting: Evidence of early death

and replacement of adipocytes. Plastic and Reconstructive Surgery. 2012;**129**:1081-1092

[16] Ferreira A d F, Gomes DA. Stem cell extracellular vesicles in skin repair. Bioengineering (Basel). 30 Dec 2018;**6**(1)

[17] Kim J-H, Jung M, Kim H-S, Kim Y-M, Choi E-H. Adipose-derived stem cells as a new therapeutic modality for ageing skin. Experimental Dermatology. 2011;**20**:383-387

[18] Zarei F, Abbaszadeh A. Stem cell and skin rejuvenation. Journal of Cosmetic and Laser Therapy. 2018;**20**:193-197

[19] Sheng L, Yang M, Liang Y, Li Q. Adipose tissue-derived stem cells (ADSCs) transplantation promotes regeneration of expanded skin using a tissue expansion model. Wound Repair and Regeneration. 2013;**21**:746-754

[20] Collawn SS, Banerjee NS, de la Torre J, Vasconez L, Chow LT. Adipose-derived stromal cells accelerate wound healing in an organotypic raft culture model. Annals of Plastic Surgery. 2012;**68**:501-504

[21] Schafer MJ, Atkinson EJ, Vanderboom PM, Kotajarvi B, White TA, Moore MM, et al. Quantification of GDF11 and myostatin in human aging and cardiovascular disease. Cell Metabolism. 2016;**23**:1207-1215

[22] Glass DJ. Elevated GDF11 is a risk factor for age-related frailty and disease in humans. Cell Metabolism. 2016;**24**:7-8

[23] Kim Y-J, Seo DH, Lee SH, Lee S-H, An G-H, Ahn H-J, et al. Conditioned media from human umbilical cord blood-derived mesenchymal stem cells stimulate rejuvenation function in human skin. Biochemistry and Biophysics Reports. 2018;**16**:96-102

[24] Idkowiak-Baldys J, Santhanam U, Buchanan SM, Pfaff KL, Rubin LL, Lyga J. Growth differentiation factor 11 (GDF11) has pronounced effects on skin biology. PLoS One. 2019;**14**:e0218035

[25] Bellei B, Migliano E, Tedesco M, Caputo S, Papaccio F, Lopez G, et al. Adipose tissue-derived extracellular fraction characterization: Biological and clinical considerations in regenerative medicine. Stem Cell Research & Therapy. 2018;**9**:207

[26] Ehrlich M, Rao J, Pabby A, Goldman MP. Improvement in the appearance of wrinkles with topical transforming growth factor beta(1) and l-ascorbic acid. Dermatologic Surgery. 2006;**32**:618-625

[27] Fisher GJ, Kang S, Varani J, Bata-Csorgo Z, Wan Y, Datta S, et al. Mechanisms of photoaging and chronological skin aging. Archives of Dermatology. 2002;**138**:1462-1470

[28] Loffredo FS, Steinhauser ML, Jay SM, Gannon J, Pancoast JR, Yalamanchi P, et al. Growth differentiation factor 11 is a circulating factor that reverses age-related cardiac hypertrophy. Cell. 2013;**153**:828-839

[29] Poggioli T, Vujic A, Yang P, Macias-Trevino C, Uygur A, Loffredo FS, et al. Circulating growth differentiation factor 11/8 levels decline with age. Circulation Research. 2016;**118**:29-37

[30] Gunin AG, Petrov VV, Golubtzova NN, Vasilieva OV, Kornilova NK. Age-related changes in angiogenesis in human dermis. Experimental Gerontology. 2014;**55**:143-151

[31] Goumans M-J, Valdimarsdottir G, Itoh S, Rosendahl A, Sideras P, ten Dijke P. Balancing the activation state of the endothelium via two distinct

TGF-beta type I receptors. The EMBO Journal. 2002;**21**:1743-1753

[32] Salvioli S, Capri M, Valensin S, Tieri P, Monti D, Ottaviani E, et al. Cytokines and aging: State of the art, new hypotheses on the role of mitochondria and new perspectives from systems biology. Current Pharmaceutical Design. 2006;**12**:3161-3171

[33] Xia S, Zhang X, Zheng S, Khanabdali R, Kalionis B, Wu J, et al. An update on inflamm-aging: Mechanisms, prevention, and treatment. Journal of Immunology Research. 2016;**2016**:8426874

[34] Bolognia JL, Cooper DL, Glusac EJ. Toxic erythema of chemotherapy: A useful clinical term. Journal of the American Academy of Dermatology. 2008;**59**:524-529

[35] Nemes Z, Steinert PM. Bricks and mortar of the epidermal barrier. Experimental & Molecular Medicine. 1999;**31**:5-19

[36] Feingold KR. The importance of lipids in cutaneous function. Journal of Lipid Research. 2007;**48**:2529-2530

[37] Smith LT, Holbrook KA, Madri JA. Collagen types I, III, and V in human embryonic and fetal skin. The American Journal of Anatomy. 1986;**175**:507-521

[38] Shin J-W, Kwon S-H, Choi J-Y, Na J-I, Huh C-H, Choi H-R, et al. Molecular mechanisms of dermal aging and antiaging approaches. International Journal of Molecular Sciences. 29 Apr 2019;**20**(9)

[39] Eckes B, Nischt R, Krieg T. Cell-matrix interactions in dermal repair and scarring. Fibrogenesis & Tissue Repair. 2010;**3**:4

[40] Giancotti FG, Ruoslahti E. Integrin signaling. Science. 1999;**285**:1028-1032

[41] Blanpain C, Fuchs E. Epidermal homeostasis: A balancing act of stem cells in the skin. Nature Reviews. Molecular Cell Biology. 2009;**10**:207-217

[42] Blanpain C, Horsley V, Fuchs E. Epithelial stem cells: Turning over new leaves. Cell. 2007;**128**:445-458

[43] Blanpain C, Fuchs E. Epidermal stem cells of the skin. Annual Review of Cell and Developmental Biology. 2006;**22**:339-373

[44] Quan T, Qin Z, Xu Y, He T, Kang S, Voorhees JJ, et al. Ultraviolet irradiation induces CYR61/CCN1, a mediator of collagen homeostasis, through activation of transcription factor AP-1 in human skin fibroblasts. The Journal of Investigative Dermatology. 2010;**130**:1697-1706

[45] Fisher GJ, Wang ZQ, Datta SC, Varani J, Kang S, Voorhees JJ. Pathophysiology of premature skin aging induced by ultraviolet light. The New England Journal of Medicine. 1997;**337**:1419-1428

[46] Varani J, Dame MK, Rittie L, Fligiel SEG, Kang S, Fisher GJ, et al. Decreased collagen production in chronologically aged skin: Roles of age-dependent alteration in fibroblast function and defective mechanical stimulation. The American Journal of Pathology. 2006;**168**:1861-1868

[47] Yang R, Fu S, Zhao L, Zhen B, Ye L, Niu X, et al. Quantitation of circulating GDF-11 and β2-MG in aged patients with age-related impairment in cognitive function. Clinical Science. 2017;**131**:1895-1904

[48] Jamaiyar A, Wan W, Janota DM, Enrick MK, Chilian WM, Yin L. The versatility and paradox of GDF 11. Pharmacology & Therapeutics. 2017;**175**:28-34

[49] Zhou Y, Jiang Z, Harris EC, Reeves J, Chen X, Pazdro R. Circulating concentrations of growth differentiation factor 11 are heritable and correlate with life span. The Journals of Gerontology. Series A, Biological Sciences and Medical Sciences. 2016;**71**:1560-1563

[50] Rochette L, Zeller M, Cottin Y, Vergely C. Growth and differentiation factor 11 (GDF11): Functions in the regulation of erythropoiesis and cardiac regeneration. Pharmacology & Therapeutics. 2015;**156**:26-33

[51] Wang Y, Wehling-Henricks M, Welc SS, Fisher AL, Zuo Q, Tidball JG. Aging of the immune system causes reductions in muscle stem cell populations, promotes their shift to a fibrogenic phenotype, and modulates sarcopenia. FASEB Journal. 2018:fj201800973R

[52] Rochette L, Meloux A, Rigal E, Zeller M, Cottin Y, Malka G, et al. Regenerative capacity of endogenous factor: Growth differentiation factor 11; a new approach of the management of age-related cardiovascular events. International Journal of Molecular Sciences. 12 Dec 2018;**19**(12)

[53] Brennan M, Bhatti H, Nerusu KC, Bhagavathula N, Kang S, Fisher GJ, et al. Matrix metalloproteinase-1 is the major collagenolytic enzyme responsible for collagen damage in UV-irradiated human skin. Photochemistry and Photobiology. 2003;**78**:43-48

[54] Patel S, Maheshwari A, Chandra A. Biomarkers for wound healing and their evaluation. Journal of Wound Care. 2016;**25**:46-55

[55] Chakraborti S, Mandal M, Das S, Mandal A, Chakraborti T. Regulation of matrix metalloproteinases: An overview. Molecular and Cellular Biochemistry. 2003;**253**:269-285

[56] Naylor EC, Watson REB, Sherratt MJ. Molecular aspects of skin ageing. Maturitas. 2011;**69**:249-256

[57] Qin Z, Balimunkwe RM, Quan T. Age-related reduction of dermal fibroblast size upregulates multiple matrix metalloproteinases as observed in aged human skin in vivo. The British Journal of Dermatology. 2017;**177**:1337-1348

[58] Pittayapruek P, Meephansan J, Prapapan O, Komine M, Ohtsuki M. Role of matrix metalloproteinases in photoaging and photocarcinogenesis. International Journal of Molecular Sciences. 2 Jun 2016;**17**(6)

[59] Lee Y, Kim H, Kim S, Kim KH, Chung JH. Activation of toll-like receptors 2, 3 or 5 induces matrix metalloproteinase-1 and -9 expression with the involvement of MAPKs and NF-kappaB in human epidermal keratinocytes. Experimental Dermatology. 2010;**19**:e44-e49

[60] Vicentini FTMC, He T, Shao Y, Fonseca MJV, Verri WA, Fisher GJ, et al. Quercetin inhibits UV irradiation-induced inflammatory cytokine production in primary human keratinocytes by suppressing NF-κB pathway. Journal of Dermatological Science. 2011;**61**:162-168

[61] Zhang Y, Lee J-H, Paull TT, Gehrke S, D'Alessandro A, Dou Q, et al. Mitochondrial redox sensing by the kinase ATM maintains cellular antioxidant capacity. Science Signaling. 10 Jul 2018;**11**(538)

[62] Newgard CB, Sharpless NE. Coming of age: Molecular drivers of aging and therapeutic opportunities. The Journal of Clinical Investigation. 2013;**123**:946-950

[63] Quan C, Cho MK, Perry D, Quan T. Age-associated reduction of

cell spreading induces mitochondrial DNA common deletion by oxidative stress in human skin dermal fibroblasts: Implication for human skin connective tissue aging. Journal of Biomedical Science. 2015;**22**:62

[64] Fisher GJ, Quan T, Purohit T, Shao Y, Cho MK, He T, et al. Collagen fragmentation promotes oxidative stress and elevates matrix metalloproteinase-1 in fibroblasts in aged human skin. The American Journal of Pathology. 2009;**174**:101-114

[65] Zorov DB, Juhaszova M, Sollott SJ. Mitochondrial reactive oxygen species (ROS) and ROS induced ROS release. Physiological Reviews. 2014;**94**:909-950

[66] Rivetti di Val Cervo P, Lena AM, Nicoloso M, Rossi S, Mancini M, Zhou H, et al. p63-microRNA feedback in keratinocyte senescence. Proceedings of the National Academy of Sciences of the United States of America. 2012;**109**:1133-1138

[67] Ressler S, Bartkova J, Niederegger H, Bartek J, Scharffetter-Kochanek K, Jansen-Dürr P, et al. p16INK4A is a robust in vivo biomarker of cellular aging in human skin. Aging Cell. 2006;**5**:379-389

[68] Nurkovic J, Volarevic V, Lako M, Armstrong L, Arsenijevic N, Stojkovic M. Aging of stem and progenitor cells: Mechanisms, impact on therapeutic potential, and rejuvenation. Rejuvenation Research. 2016;**19**:3-12

[69] Barrientos S, Stojadinovic O, Golinko MS, Brem H, Tomic-Canic M. Growth factors and cytokines in wound healing. Wound Repair and Regeneration. 2008;**16**:585-601

[70] Hur W, Lee HY, Min HS, Wufuer M, Lee C-W, Hur JA, et al. Regeneration of full-thickness skin defects by differentiated adipose-derived stem cells into fibroblast-like cells by fibroblast-conditioned medium. Stem Cell Research & Therapy. 2017;**8**:92

[71] Komaki M, Numata Y, Morioka C, Honda I, Tooi M, Yokoyama N, et al. Exosomes of human placenta-derived mesenchymal stem cells stimulate angiogenesis. Stem Cell Research & Therapy. 2017;**8**:219

[72] Bachmann S, Jennewein M, Bubel M, Guthörl S, Pohlemann T, Oberringer M. Interacting adipose-derived stem cells and microvascular endothelial cells provide a beneficial milieu for soft tissue healing. Molecular Biology Reports. Jan 2020;**47**(1):111-122

[73] Lynch SE, Nixon JC, Colvin RB, Antoniades HN. Role of platelet-derived growth factor in wound healing: Synergistic effects with other growth factors. Proceedings of the National Academy of Sciences of the United States of America. 1987;**84**:7696-7700

[74] Park B-S, Jang KA, Sung J-H, Park J-S, Kwon YH, Kim KJ, et al. Adipose-derived stem cells and their secretory factors as a promising therapy for skin aging. Dermatologic Surgery. 2008;**34**:1323-1326

[75] Pierce GF, Mustoe TA, Lingelbach J, Masakowski VR, Griffin GL, Senior RM, et al. Platelet-derived growth factor and transforming growth factor-beta enhance tissue repair activities by unique mechanisms. The Journal of Cell Biology. 1989;**109**:429-440

[76] Gonzalo-Daganzo R, Regidor C, Martín-Donaire T, Rico MA, Bautista G, Krsnik I, et al. Results of a pilot study on the use of third-party donor mesenchymal stromal cells in cord blood transplantation in adults. Cytotherapy. 2009;**11**:278-288

[77] Ucuzian AA, Gassman AA, East AT, Greisler HP. Molecular mediators of

angiogenesis. Journal of Burn Care & Research. 2010;**31**:158-175

[78] Sumi M, Sata M, Toya N, Yanaga K, Ohki T, Nagai R. Transplantation of adipose stromal cells, but not mature adipocytes, augments ischemia-induced angiogenesis. Life Sciences. 2007;**80**:559-565

[79] Liu Y, Cox SR, Morita T, Kourembanas S. Hypoxia regulates vascular endothelial growth factor gene expression in endothelial cells. Identification of a 5′ enhancer. Circulation Research. 1995;**77**:638-643

[80] Romaldini A, Mastrogiacomo M, Cancedda R, Descalzi F. Platelet lysate activates human subcutaneous adipose tissue cells by promoting cell proliferation and their paracrine activity toward epidermal keratinocytes. Frontiers in Bioengineering and Biotechnology. 2018;**6**:203

[81] Caley MP, Martins VLC, O'Toole EA. Metalloproteinases and wound healing. Advances in Wound Care (New Rochelle). 2015;**4**:225-234

[82] Seppanen E, Roy E, Ellis R, Bou-Gharios G, Fisk NM, Khosrotehrani K. Distant mesenchymal progenitors contribute to skin wound healing and produce collagen: Evidence from a murine fetal microchimerism model. PLoS One. 2013;**8**:e62662

[83] Waterman RS, Tomchuck SL, Henkle SL, Betancourt AM. A new mesenchymal stem cell (MSC) paradigm: Polarization into a pro-inflammatory MSC1 or an immunosuppressive MSC2 phenotype. PLoS One. 2010;**5**:e10088

[84] Park JE, Barbul A. Understanding the role of immune regulation in wound healing. American Journal of Surgery. 2004;**187**:11S-16S

[85] Anderson PH. Vitamin D activity and metabolism in bone. Current Osteoporosis Reports. 2017;**15**:443-449

[86] Baharlou R, Ahmadi-Vasmehjani A, Faraji F, Atashzar MR, Khoubyari M, Ahi S, et al. Human adipose tissue-derived mesenchymal stem cells in rheumatoid arthritis: Regulatory effects on peripheral blood mononuclear cells activation. International Immunopharmacology. 2017;**47**:59-69

[87] Lozito TP, Jackson WM, Nesti LJ, Tuan RS. Human mesenchymal stem cells generate a distinct pericellular zone of MMP activities via binding of MMPs and secretion of high levels of TIMPs. Matrix Biology. 2014;**34**:132-143

[88] Xiao W, Tang H, Wu M, Liao Y, Li K, Li L, et al. Ozone oil promotes wound healing by increasing the migration of fibroblasts via PI3K/Akt/mTOR signaling pathway. Bioscience Reports. 2017;**37**

[89] Koivisto L, Bi J, Häkkinen L, Larjava H. Integrin αvβ6: Structure, function and role in health and disease. The International Journal of Biochemistry & Cell Biology. 2018;**99**:186-196

[90] Ferreira A d F, Cunha PS, Carregal VM, da Silva PC, de Miranda MC, Kunrath-Lima M, et al. Extracellular vesicles from adipose-derived mesenchymal stem/stromal cells accelerate migration and activate AKT pathway in human keratinocytes and fibroblasts independently of miR-205 activity. Stem Cells International. 2017;**2017**:9841035

[91] Rehman J, Traktuev D, Li J, Merfeld-Clauss S, Temm-Grove CJ, Bovenkerk JE, et al. Secretion of angiogenic and antiapoptotic factors by human adipose stromal cells. Circulation. 2004;**109**:1292-1298

[92] Planat-Benard V, Silvestre J-S, Cousin B, André M, Nibbelink M, Tamarat R, et al. Plasticity of human adipose lineage cells toward endothelial cells: Physiological and therapeutic

perspectives. Circulation. 2004;**109**:656-663

[93] Sasaki M, Abe R, Fujita Y, Ando S, Inokuma D, Shimizu H. Mesenchymal stem cells are recruited into wounded skin and contribute to wound repair by transdifferentiation into multiple skin cell type. Journal of Immunology. 2008;**180**:2581-2587

[94] Zimmers TA, Jiang Y, Wang M, Liang TW, Rupert JE, Au ED, et al. Exogenous GDF11 induces cardiac and skeletal muscle dysfunction and wasting. Basic Research in Cardiology. 2017;**112**:48

[95] Tito A, Barbulova A, Zappelli C, Leone M, Ruvo M, Mercurio FA, et al. The growth differentiation factor 11 is involved in skin fibroblast ageing and is induced by a preparation of peptides and sugars derived from plant cell cultures. Molecular Biotechnology. 2019;**61**:209-220

[96] Dabiri G, Campaner A, Morgan JR, Van De Water L. A TGF-beta1-dependent autocrine loop regulates the structure of focal adhesions in hypertrophic scar fibroblasts. The Journal of Investigative Dermatology. 2006;**126**:963-970

[97] Mohan R, Chintala SK, Jung JC, Villar WVL, McCabe F, Russo LA, et al. Matrix metalloproteinase gelatinase B (MMP-9) coordinates and effects epithelial regeneration. The Journal of Biological Chemistry. 2002;**277**:2065-2072

[98] Rennert RC et al. Stem cell recruitment after injury: Lessons for regenerative medicine. Regenerative Medicine. PubMed – NCBI. Available from: https://www.ncbi.nlm.nih.gov/pubmed/23164083 [Accessed: 19 November 2019]

[99] Ji F, Wang Y, Yuan J, Wu Q, Wang J, Liu D. The potential role of stromal cell-derived factor-1α/CXCR4/CXCR7 axis in adipose-derived mesenchymal stem cells. Journal of Cellular Physiology. Apr 2020;**235**(4):3548-3557

[100] Klar AS, Zimoch J, Biedermann T. Skin tissue engineering: Application of adipose-derived stem cells. BioMed Research International. 2017;**2017**:9747010

[101] Wang Y, Viennet C, Robin S, Berthon J-Y, He L, Humbert P. Precise role of dermal fibroblasts on melanocyte pigmentation. Journal of Dermatological Science. 2017;**88**:159-166

[102] Höhn A, Weber D, Jung T, Ott C, Hugo M, Kochlik B, et al. Happily (n)ever after: Aging in the context of oxidative stress, proteostasis loss and cellular senescence. Redox Biology. 2017;**11**:482-501

[103] Qin S, Zheng J-H, Xia Z-H, Qian J, Deng C-L, Yang S-L. CTHRC1 promotes wound repair by increasing M2 macrophages via regulating the TGF-β and notch pathways. Biomedicine & Pharmacotherapy. 2019;**113**:108594

[104] Revu S, Wu J, Henkel M, Rittenhouse N, Menk A, Delgoffe GM, et al. IL-23 and IL-1β drive human Th17 cell differentiation and metabolic reprogramming in absence of CD28 costimulation. Cell Reports. 2018;**22**:2642-2653

[105] Mei W, Xiang G, Li Y, Li H, Xiang L, Lu J, et al. GDF11 protects against endothelial injury and reduces atherosclerotic lesion formation in apolipoprotein E-null mice. Molecular Therapy. 2016;**24**:1926-1938

[106] Das T, Chen Z, Hendriks RW, Kool M. A20/tumor necrosis factor α-induced protein 3 in immune cells controls development of autoinflammation and autoimmunity: Lessons from mouse models. Frontiers in Immunology. 2018;**9**:104

[107] Othmani AE, Rouam S, Abbad A, Erraoui C, Harriba S, Boukind H, et al. Cryopreservation impacts cell functionality of long term expanded adipose-derived stem cells. Journal of Stem Cell Research & Therapy. 2019;**9**:445

[108] Kim W-S, Park B-S, Sung J-H. Protective role of adipose-derived stem cells and their soluble factors in photoaging. Archives of Dermatological Research. 2009;**301**:329-336

[109] Niada S, Giannasi C, Gualerzi A, Banfi G, Brini AT. Differential proteomic analysis predicts appropriate applications for the secretome of adipose-derived mesenchymal stem/stromal cells and dermal fibroblasts. Stem Cells International. 2018;**2018**:7309031

[110] Hu L, Wang J, Zhou X, Xiong Z, Zhao J, Yu R, et al. Exosomes derived from human adipose mensenchymal stem cells accelerates cutaneous wound healing via optimizing the characteristics of fibroblasts. Scientific Reports. 2016;**6**:32993

[111] Wang T, Guo S, Liu X, Xv N, Zhang S. Protective effects of adipose-derived stem cells secretome on human dermal fibroblasts from ageing damages. International Journal of Clinical and Experimental Pathology. 2015;**8**:15739-15748

[112] Gaur M, Dobke M, Lunyak VV. Mesenchymal stem cells from adipose tissue in clinical applications for dermatological indications and skin aging. International Journal of Molecular Sciences. 20 Jan 2017;**18**(1)

[113] Son W-C, Yun J-W, Kim B-H. Adipose-derived mesenchymal stem cells reduce MMP-1 expression in UV-irradiated human dermal fibroblasts: Therapeutic potential in skin wrinkling. Bioscience, Biotechnology, and Biochemistry. 2015;**79**:919-925

[114] Na YK, Ban J-J, Lee M, Im W, Kim M. Wound healing potential of adipose tissue stem cell extract. Biochemical and Biophysical Research Communications. 2017;**485**:30-34

[115] Ma N, Qiao C, Zhang W, Luo H, Zhang X, Liu D, et al. Original research: Adipose-derived stem cells from younger donors, but not aging donors, inspire the host self-healing capability through its secreta. Experimental Biology and Medicine (Maywood, N.J.). 2017;**242**:68-79

[116] Bueno JL, Ynigo M, de Miguel C, Gonzalo-Daganzo RM, Richart A, Vilches C, et al. Growth differentiation factor 11 (GDF11)—A promising anti-ageing factor—Is highly concentrated in platelets. Vox Sanguinis. 2016;**111**:434-436

[117] Tooi M, Komaki M, Morioka C, Honda I, Iwasaki K, Yokoyama N, et al. Placenta mesenchymal stem cell derived exosomes confer plasticity on fibroblasts. Journal of Cellular Biochemistry. 2016;**117**:1658-1670

[118] Kim H-S, Lee JH, Roh K-H, Jun HJ, Kang K-S, Kim T-Y. Clinical trial of human umbilical cord blood-derived stem cells for the treatment of moderate-to-severe atopic dermatitis: Phase I/IIa studies. Stem Cells. 2017;**35**:248-255

[119] Zografou A, Tsigris C, Papadopoulos O, Kavantzas N, Patsouris E, Donta I, et al. Improvement of skin-graft survival after autologous transplantation of adipose-derived stem cells in rats. Journal of Plastic, Reconstructive & Aesthetic Surgery. 2011;**64**:1647-1656

[120] Kim W-S, Park B-S, Kim H-K, Park J-S, Kim K-J, Choi J-S, et al. Evidence supporting antioxidant action of adipose-derived stem cells: Protection of human dermal fibroblasts from oxidative stress.

Journal of Dermatological Science. 2008;**49**:133-142

[121] Phelps J, Sanati-Nezhad A, Ungrin M, Duncan NA, Sen A. Bioprocessing of mesenchymal stem cells and their derivatives: Toward cell-free therapeutics. Stem Cells International. 2018;**2018**:9415367

[122] Kobayashi T, Kim H, Liu X, Sugiura H, Kohyama T, Fang Q, et al. Matrix metalloproteinase-9 activates TGF-β and stimulates fibroblast contraction of collagen gels. American Journal of Physiology. Lung Cellular and Molecular Physiology. 2014;**306**:L1006-L1015

[123] Wang AS, Dreesen O. Biomarkers of cellular senescence and skin aging. Frontiers in Genetics. 2018;**9**:247

[124] Lunyak VV, Amaro-Ortiz A, Gaur M. Mesenchymal stem cells secretory responses: Senescence messaging secretome and immunomodulation perspective. Frontiers in Genetics. 2017;**8**:220

[125] Lee S-H, Lee J-H, Lee H-Y, Min K-J. Sirtuin signaling in cellular senescence and aging. BMB Reports. 2019;**52**:24-34

[126] Tigges J, Krutmann J, Fritsche E, Haendeler J, Schaal H, Fischer JW, et al. The hallmarks of fibroblast ageing. Mechanisms of Ageing and Development. 2014;**138**:26-44

[127] Singh CK, Chhabra G, Ndiaye MA, Garcia-Peterson LM, Mack NJ, Ahmad N. The role of sirtuins in antioxidant and redox signaling. Antioxidants & Redox Signaling. 2018;**28**:643-661

[128] Garcia-Peterson LM, Wilking-Busch MJ, Ndiaye MA, Philippe CGA, Setaluri V, Ahmad N. Sirtuins in skin and skin cancers. Skin Pharmacology and Physiology. 2017;**30**:216-224

[129] Goyarts EC, Dong K, Pelle E, Pernodet N. Effect of SIRT6 knockdown on NF-κB induction and on residual DNA damage in cultured human skin fibroblasts. Journal of Cosmetic Science. 2017;**68**:25-33

[130] Jun EK, Zhang Q, Yoon BS, Moon J-H, Lee G, Park G, et al. Hypoxic conditioned medium from human amniotic fluid-derived mesenchymal stem cells accelerates skin wound healing through TGF-β/SMAD2 and PI3K/Akt pathways. International Journal of Molecular Sciences. 2014;**15**:605-628

[131] Fang X, Hu X, Zheng Z, Tao K, Wang H, Guan H, et al. Smad interacting protein 1 influences transforming growth factor-β1/Smad signaling in extracellular matrix protein production and hypertrophic scar formation. Journal of Molecular Histology. 2019;**50**:503-514

[132] Fang S, Xu C, Zhang Y, Xue C, Yang C, Bi H, et al. Umbilical cord-derived mesenchymal stem cell-derived exosomal microRNAs suppress myofibroblast differentiation by inhibiting the transforming growth factor-β/SMAD2 pathway during wound healing. Stem Cells Translational Medicine. 2016;**5**:1425-1439

[133] Luo H, Guo Y, Liu Y, Wang Y, Zheng R, Ban Y, et al. Growth differentiation factor 11 inhibits adipogenic differentiation by activating TGF-beta/Smad signalling pathway. Cell Proliferation. 2019;**52**:e12631

[134] Lu Q, Tu M-L, Li C-J, Zhang L, Jiang T-J, Liu T, et al. GDF11 inhibits bone formation by activating Smad2/3 in bone marrow mesenchymal stem cells. Calcified Tissue International. 2016;**99**:500-509

[135] Rivera-Gonzalez GC, Shook BA, Andrae J, Holtrup B, Bollag K, Betsholtz C, et al. Skin adipocyte stem

cell self-renewal is regulated by a PDGFA/AKT-signaling axis. Cell Stem Cell. 2016;**19**:738-751

[136] Walter MNM, Wright KT, Fuller HR, MacNeil S, Johnson WEB. Mesenchymal stem cell-conditioned medium accelerates skin wound healing: An in vitro study of fibroblast and keratinocyte scratch assays. Experimental Cell Research. 2010;**316**:1271-1281

[137] Bose B, Shenoy PS. Pluripotent conversion of muscle stem cells without reprogramming factors or small molecules. Stem Cell Reviews and Reports. 2016;**12**:73-89

[138] Houschyar KS, Momeni A, Pyles MN, Maan ZN, Whittam AJ, Siemers F. Wnt signaling induces epithelial differentiation during cutaneous wound healing. Organogenesis. 2015;**11**:95-104

[139] Maddaluno L, Urwyler C, Werner S. Fibroblast growth factors: Key players in regeneration and tissue repair. Development. 2017;**144**:4047-4060

[140] de Araújo R, Lôbo M, Trindade K, Silva DF, Pereira N. Fibroblast growth factors: A controlling mechanism of skin aging. Skin Pharmacology and Physiology. 2019;**32**:275-282

[141] Baumann L. Skin ageing and its treatment. The Journal of Pathology. 2007;**211**:241-251

[142] Żerańska J, Pasikowska M, Szczepanik B, Mlosek K, Malinowska S, Dębowska RM, et al. A study of the activity and effectiveness of recombinant fibroblast growth factor (Q40P/S47I/H93G rFGF-1) in anti-aging treatment. Postepy Dermatologii I Alergologii. 2016;**33**:28-36

[143] Zakrzewska M, Krowarsch D, Wiedlocha A, Otlewski J. Design of fully active FGF-1 variants with increased stability. Protein Engineering, Design & Selection. 2004;**17**:603-611

[144] Weiss RA, Weiss MA. Evaluation of a novel anti-aging topical formulation containing cycloastragenol, growth factors, peptides, and antioxidants. Journal of Drugs in Dermatology. 2014;**13**:1135-1139

[145] Yang L, Zhang D, Wu H, Xie S, Zhang M, Zhang B, et al. Basic fibroblast growth factor influences epidermal homeostasis of living skin equivalents through affecting fibroblast phenotypes and functions. Skin Pharmacology and Physiology. 2018;**31**:229-237

[146] Acosta JC, Banito A, Wuestefeld T, Georgilis A, Janich P, Morton JP, et al. A complex secretory program orchestrated by the inflammasome controls paracrine senescence. Nature Cell Biology. 2013;**15**:978-990

Chapter 3

Isolation, Activation, and Mechanism of Action of Platelet-Rich Plasma and Its Applications for Joint Repair

Mikel Sánchez, Maider Beitia, Orlando Pompei, Cristina Jorquera, Pello Sánchez, Jorge Knörr, Francisco Soldado, Leonor López, Jaime Oraa, Ane Miren Bilbao, Nicolás Fiz, Jorge Guadilla, Beatriz Aizpurua, Juan Azofra and Diego Delgado

Abstract

Platelet-Rich Plasma (PRP) is a biologic therapy that uses the patient's own blood to obtain products with a higher platelet concentration than in blood. This technology provides a controlled drug delivery system of growth factors suitable for regenerative medicine. The biological effects of PRP mimic and influence biological processes such as inflammation, analgesia, and cell stimulation, providing this therapy with promising therapeutic potential. All these processes participate in maintenance, correct function, and homeostasis of the joint, where all tissues are involved. Alterations in one joint element have impact on the rest, outstanding the cellular and molecular interaction between the cartilage and subchondral bone. Therefore, the joint is an optimal therapeutic target for PRP therapy, which favors biological environment for joint repair. This chapter collects the basic concepts of joint function and the biological processes that participate in its degeneration, the definition and obtention of PRP, as well as its therapeutic potential and clinical translation.

Keywords: Platelet-Rich Plasma, growth factors, joint degeneration, cartilage, subchondral bone, intra-articular injection, intraosseous injection

1. Introduction

Despite joint degeneration, caused mainly by osteoarthritis (OA), not being a threat to life, it meets conditions that make it a real problem for both patients and health systems. This pathology is one of the leading causes of disability in the middle-aged and elderly population, and although any joint can be affected, the hip and knee are the most affected ones. This high prevalence, with 250 million people with knee OA throughout the world, represents up to 2.5% of gross domestic product for developed countries [1]. In the coming years, prevalence and costs will increase because the risk factors that favor OA are inherent to today's society such as the aging of the population, overweight, or an uncontrolled sports practice, both by excess and by default.

Patients with OA are characterized by pain, stiffness, and limitation of function, becoming disabling in the most advanced stages [2]. Initial conservative treatments include physiotherapeutic work, nutritional supplements, and oral administration of analgesic and anti-inflammatories. In the next phases, patients can be treated with intra-articular injections of hyaluronic acid. Regardless of the success of these treatments, all of them focus on symptomatic relief without stopping or slowing the progression of the disease, and the only solution for patients with the most severe degrees of OA is total knee arthroplasty [3]. This surgical intervention not only entails the risks derived from surgery, which may be unacceptable by some patients, but also involves the majority of the cost of health systems [4, 5]. Therefore, it is necessary to develop new therapies that improve the current ones in order not only to alleviate the symptoms but also to modify the course of the pathology to slow its progression or even reverse it. This would improve the quality of life of patients, delaying or avoiding a large number of surgical interventions as well as the expense they entail.

These therapies must be based on two main pillars that sustain a new approach in joint degeneration: first, treatments based on regenerative medicine which can act on tissue biology and modify the pathophysiology of OA such as gene therapy, Platelet-Rich Plasma (PRP), or mesenchymal stem cells (MSCs). Among these treatments, PRP is currently the most widely used due to its greater ease of regulating, obtaining, and applying as well as its low cost [6, 7]. However, it is necessary to deepen their knowledge and standardize products and protocols to optimize clinical results. The second cornerstone is to understand the joint as a whole organ, taking into consideration all its elements [8]. Knowing the relationships between the different tissues that form and define the joint is key for the correct application of treatments and address degenerative pathology completely. Thus, this chapter is intended to explain the role of PRP in joint degeneration, highlighting the therapeutic potential of PRP in all the components of the joint and its clinical translation.

2. The joint as an organ

2.1 Joint components and homeostasis maintenance

All joint structures present a unique molecular and cellular composition as well as specific biomechanical properties; consequently, each element of the joint performs characteristic functions. However, they are all coordinated and related to create the biological machinery that allows the joint to have dynamic stability (**Figure 1**) [9]. This gives the joint a great adaptability to maintain a mechanical and biological balance, supporting and confronting physical forces or physiologic disorders. In a short look at the components of the joint, the periarticular muscles appear in the outermost section. This tissue presents vascular irrigation, many neuronal terminals, and high plasticity. The configuration of its extracellular matrix in a network of muscle fibers provides muscle elasticity and allows the mechanical forces generated by the muscle cells to be transmitted to the tendons, which will translate them into joint mobility [10]. However, its stability capacity is even more important than mobility in order to maintain joint homeostasis, the quadriceps muscle being key in knee anteroposterior steadiness. In addition, muscle tissue is essential in shock-absorbing, and together with the subchondral bone and ligaments, it accounts for 30–50% of the total absorbing energy [11]. Ligament composition is characterized by a high-water content and an extracellular matrix with

DOI: http://dx.doi.org/10.5772/intechopen.90543

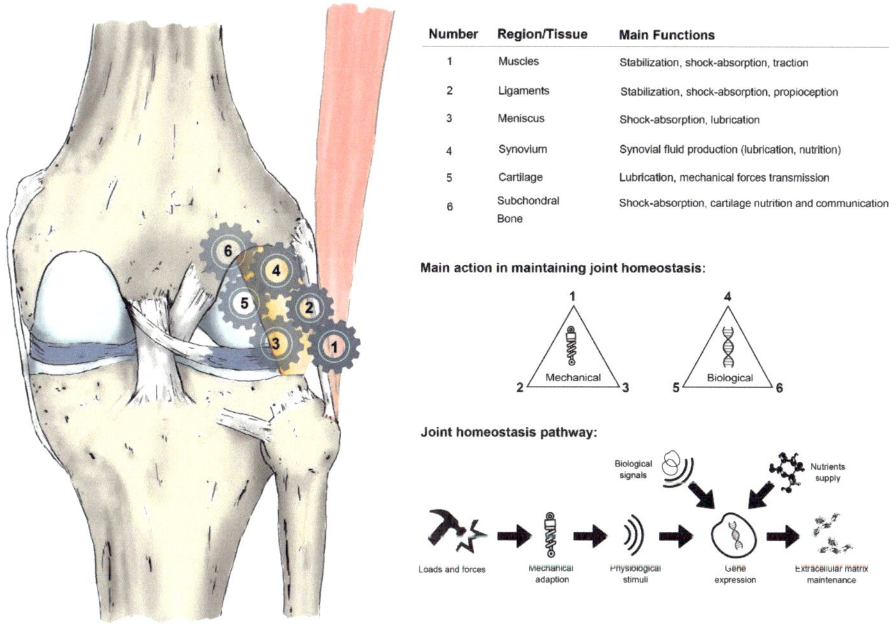

Figure 1.
Joint as an organ. All the elements of the joint participate in its correct function and in the maintenance of the homeostasis. Although they all contribute to mechanical and biological stabilization, ligament and meniscus muscles play a mainly mechanical role, whereas the synovium, cartilage, and subchondral bone have a more biological action. Correct mechanical adaptation and a favorable biological environment allow the cells to maintain a gene expression that promotes the optimal maintenance of the extracellular matrix.

a small number of fibroblasts. Collagen is the most predominant protein, mainly organized in type I collagen fibers that adopt many directions and orientations due to several forces these structures are subjected to [12]. Apart from their stabilizing function due to their biomechanical and viscoelastic properties, they are also responsible for detecting and controlling the position and movement of the knee. In this way, the joint has a balanced biomechanical behavior that prevents the origin of mechanical problems that lead to degeneration. The meniscus plays a fundamental role in functions of mechanical nature such as stability and shock-absorbing. It is a fibrocartilaginous tissue with an abundant extracellular matrix where cells such as fibroblasts and fibrochondrocytes are dispersed and where type I collagen is the predominant molecule. The presence of vascularization and nerve terminals is limited to the external zone or meniscal wall. These intra-articular elements located between the femoral condyles and the tibial plateau help stabilize the joint and withstand compression and sharing forces. In addition, they participate in the lubrication of the joint with the synovial membrane or synovium [13].

The synovium, together with the cartilage and subchondral bone, forms an important biological triangle to maintain homeostasis of the knee. Both nerve fibers and blood vessels are abundant in the synovium, which provides nutrients not only to this structure but also to the adjacent avascular cartilage. Its cellular composition stands out mainly for synoviocytes (macrophagic cells or type A and fibroblast-like cells or type B), although immune system cells and even MSCs are also present, the synovium being a source of stem cells of increasing interest [14]. Its main function is the production of synovial fluid, which is produced by type B synoviocytes. It soaks the intra-articular space and structures, being essential in the lubrication of the joint due to its hyaluronic acid and lubricin content. The synovial fluid is also an important source of nutrients, biomolecules, and cellular signals, so it is essential for the biological balance of the joint [15]. The second element of this biological triangle is the hyaline articular cartilage. It has a very low coefficient of friction that resists compression and shear forces and absorbs only 1–3% of the total energy. The main cellular element of this tissue is a low population of chondrocytes that is distributed along the extracellular matrix composed principally of type 2 collagen, in addition to other molecules such as proteoglycans or aggrecans. Its functions of lubrication and transmission of mechanical forces are performed thanks to a stratified tissue in different zones, from the most superficial, with a higher water content and chondrocytes, to a deeper area of calcified cartilage that is over the subchondral bone [16].

Subchondral bone, together with the osteochondral unit, completes the triad of elements with a predominant role in the biological maintenance of the joint. This structure consists of a plate of cortical bone from where the bone marrow and trabecular bone areas emerge. The importance of the subchondral bone lies in its communication with the cartilage, providing this tissue with at least 50% of the oxygen and glucose requirements. This communication not only is limited to the nutritional contribution but also covers the cellular and molecular signaling that participates in the cartilage homeostasis. Besides this, it is also a source of MSCs and participates in absorbing joint loads along with the other elements mentioned above [17].

The joint adaptability is both mechanical and biological, and it is in this last component where the action of regenerative medicine could positively influence. All the structures and tissues described above participate in joint stability by adapting to the different alterations and stimuli received, ultimately maintaining a healthy cartilage. Because of the "mechanical stabilizers" of the joint, the mechanical loads and forces that it receives become molecular and cellular stimuli that are maintained at physiological levels. These stimuli activate the chondrocyte gene expression, allowing them to synthesize proteins, such as proteoglycans, collagen, and metalloproteases, that ensure the integrity and renovation of the articular cartilage [18]. The continuous adaptation of the cells to the mechanical stimuli they receive in order to maintain the adequate extracellular matrix is based on a very delicate anabolic/catabolic balance, and any mechanical or biological alteration can break it resulting in joint degeneration [19].

2.2 Joint degeneration process

The balance present in the joint may be broken because of multiple causes (**Figure 2**). For example, injuries of the tissues involved in the mechanical stabilization of the knee could entail an abnormal load distribution. This would cause an unsatisfactory shock absorption into the joint, and the stimuli generated would exceed the physiological level [20]. Lifestyle can also have an impact on the generation of pathological stimuli. Both uncontrolled physical activity and sedentary lifestyle lead to an excess or defect of stimuli, respectively. The result is a biological and cellular malfunction and, consequently, a defective tissue renewal. In addition, pathologies and biological disorders such as inflammatory processes or those affecting the structures responsible for maintaining and nourishing the cartilage could also cause cellular failures that lead to imbalance and joint degeneration.

The multifactorial nature of this pathology makes it difficult to know the exact origin of the triggered processes as well as their sequence and timing. These events take place with special importance in the interaction between the synovial membrane, cartilage, and subchondral bone. Regardless of the original cause, one of the main consequences of this imbalance is the deterioration of the extracellular matrix and the generation of degradation products that are released to the synovial fluid [21]. The cells of the different joint tissues such as chondrocytes, synovial macrophages, osteoblasts, or fibroblast interact with these molecules, which act as Toll-like-receptors (TLRs) and damage-associated molecular patterns (DAMPs).

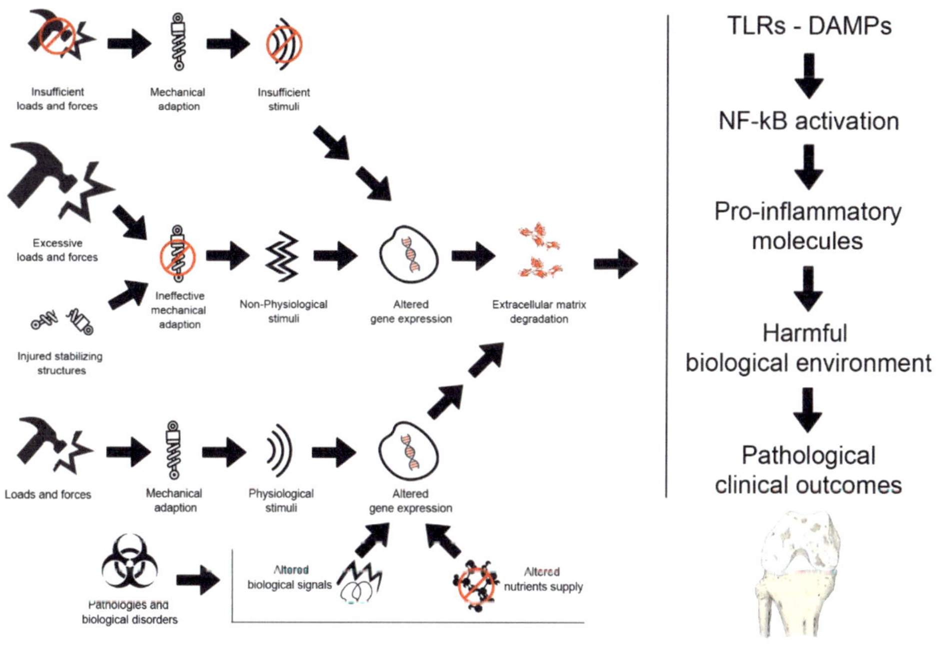

Figure 2.
Joint degeneration processes. Different causes such as abnormal mechanical loads, injuries of stabilizing structures, or pathologies and biological disorders cause nonphysiological stimuli that modify the gene expression of cells. As a consequence, the extracellular matrix degenerates, activating pro-inflammatory pathways that create a harmful environment and joint degeneration.

As a consequence of these interactions, the intracellular pathway of the nuclear factor kappa β (NF-kB) is activated, connecting the mechanobiological program and the inflammatory response. The gene expression of the affected cells shifts to an inflammatory pattern synthesizing molecules, namely, interleukins (IL-1b, IL-6, IL10), prostaglandins (PEG-2) and other pro-inflammatory biomolecules, and cytokines (necrosis factor alpha (TNF-α), interferon gamma, or nerve growth factor (NGF)). Pathological levels of these molecules also interfere in physiological repairing responses. For instance, the action of MSCs from the bone marrow is altered by high levels of transforming growth factor beta (TGF-β), compromising their modulating and repairing functions [22].

All the harmful biological environment generated by this event cascade leads to pathological outcomes in the cartilage, synovium, and subchondral bone. Chondrocytes of cartilage turn into a much more active state, forming cell clusters and increasing their proliferation. They also increase the synthesis of both extracellular matrix proteins and enzymes, causing an altered remodeling of the matrix with hypertrophy and calcifications [19]. Concerning the synovium, inflammation occurs in the early stages together with macrophage infiltrates and an increased synovitis in the advanced stages [23]. Communications between the cartilage and subchondral bone are increased due to the presence of fissures and microcraks, in addition to the remodeling of this tissue with fibroneuroangiogenesis because of the overexpression of molecules like TGF-β and vascular endothelial growth factor (VEGF) [24].

Moreover, the negative effects arising from joint degeneration can affect other tissues as well [8]. For example, studies conducted in the meniscus of patients with arthrosis showed a tissue with increased vascularization and nerve terminals, with the unstructured extracellular matrix, abnormal cell organization, and cell death [25]. Likewise, ligaments with osteoarthritic patients also showed calcifications and disorganized collagen fibers [26]. Finally, muscle tissue is also affected by inflammation produced in joint degeneration, showing fibrosis, collagen depositions, and muscle wasting [27]. Considering all this, it is clear that joint degeneration is not a sole cartilage disease. Instead, it affects all the elements present in the joint, and, therefore, it should be clinically tackled taking into consideration all of them in order to reverse or slow down the degenerative progression.

3. Platelet-Rich Plasma

3.1 Platelets as a source of bioactive molecules

PRP is an autologous biological therapy framed in the regenerative medicine whose basic principle is to obtain a fraction of blood plasma that contains platelets at a higher concentration than in the blood. From the pharmacological perspective, it is very difficult to define it since the PRP presents a large number and variety of active substances, even often antagonistic. Its therapeutic potential lies both in the biomolecules present in the plasma and in the platelet and its content that is the core element of this therapy.

The platelets are produced by the megakaryocytes of the bone marrow, which migrate to the endothelial barrier after maturation and project their prolongations releasing into the bloodstream the proplatelets or precursors that will generate the platelets [28]. Platelets are discoid and anucleated blood elements with a diameter of 2–3 μm; their blood concentration is 150.000–400.000 platelets/μL with a life span of 7 to 10 days. Platelets are limited by an external plasma membrane that contains a large network of receptors that trigger intracellular signals that allow platelets to perform their numerous functions. Among them glycoprotein Ib (GPiB) and glycoprotein VI (GPVI) receptors can be found, which are involved in functions related to homeostasis, the main function of platelets. GPIb and GPVI bind to von Willebrand factor (VWF) and collagen when there is a discontinuity in the endothelial barrier that exposes the extracellular matrix. These interactions cause conformational changes in platelets and allow them to bind to fibrinogen, tissues, and other platelets to form the thrombus that will participate in tissue repair. In addition, this platelet activation also causes the release of their internal content that has regenerative abilities and justifies the use of PRP.

The internal content of platelets is stored in different granules called dense granules, α-granules, and lysosomes. The material present in these granules may have been synthesized by the original megakaryocyte as well as captured by platelets by endocytosis. The α-granules are those that have a higher content of active biomolecules related to tissue repair. Hundreds of these molecules have been identified, including adhesive proteins, fibrinolytic and coagulation factors, antimicrobial molecules, cytokines, and growth factors, among others. These last two groups of molecules participate in tissue repair and regeneration processes such as angiogenesis, chemotaxis, migration, or cell proliferation [29]. When platelets are activated, not only these molecules are released but also other elements such as platelet microparticles, which are involved in anti-inflammatory processes, or exosomes. Exosomes are small vesicles of 100–400 nm that carry several proteins in addition to other biomolecules as genetic material. Although not much is known about these platelet exosomes, it has been found that they are very important in cellular communication [30].

The activation of the PRP platelets causes the release of platelet content related to tissue repair to the outside, and it joins to the circulating biomolecules in the plasma. Thus, the levels of many growth factors will depend on the platelet concentration of the PRP. Among these platelet growth factors, there is platelet-derived growth factor (PDGF), which is a potent chemotactic for several cell types and has an important effect on tissue repair over tissues such as cartilage and meniscus. Another growth factor with a large presence in platelets is TGF-β, whose effects are varied and can be of different nature depending on the molecules and cells with which it interacts. It influences early responses in tissue repair, on the differentiation processes of mesenchymal stem cells, and on the maintenance of cartilage and subchondral bone. Other regulatory factors in tissue repair are VEGF, epidermal growth factor (EGF), or basic fibroblast growth factor (bFGF) with key roles in cell migration, proliferation, differentiation, or angiogenesis. In addition, circulating molecules such as insulin-like growth factor type I (IGF-I) or hepatocyte growth factor (HGF) have also crucial importance in the effect of PRP; they are growth factor enhancers of regeneration processes as well as modulators of inflammatory processes [31].

Therefore, PRP is a cocktail of thousands of biomolecules from plasma and platelets that regulate hemostasis, coagulation, tissue repair and regeneration, inflammation, cellular behavior, or defense against microorganisms, among other biological processes. All this therapeutic potential depends largely on its composition, which may vary according to the method used to obtain it. As a result, there is a wide variety of PRP products as will be explained below.

3.2 Obtaining process

3.2.1 Blood collection

As stated previously, the PRP obtaining technique is used to achieve a fraction of blood plasma with higher levels of platelets than blood. The first step consists in the collection of a small volume of peripheral blood from the patient using tubes with anticoagulant—to prevent blood clotting. Different types of anticoagulants can be used such as sodium citrate and ethylenediaminetetraacetic acid (EDTA), which chelate calcium and prevent the coagulation cascade, or heparin that inhibits thrombin. However, sodium citrate is the most recommended anticoagulant since it ensures a better preservation of platelets [32]. It also causes less secretion of microvesicles that are the result of platelet activation, which is increased when EDTA and heparin are used as blood anticoagulants [33].

3.2.2 Blood fractionation and Platelet-Rich Plasma obtention

After blood collection, a centrifugation process is performed, whose force and time vary according to the methodology and, hence, the PRP formulation to be obtained. Centrifugation has to generate sufficient force to create a gradient that separates the blood into different fractions but without damaging its components (**Figure 3**). These centrifugations can be single or double, with a centrifugal force of between 350 and 2000 g and a centrifugation time of 3 to 15 minutes depending on the method used. Thus, the blood is divided into a lower fraction of red blood cells, a thin layer of leukocytes or buffy coat, and finally the plasma fraction with platelets, which gradually decrease their number in the uppermost areas. This last layer will constitute the PRP, and depending on the centrifugation process, the number of platelets may vary. However, a higher number of platelets are not strictly linked to an improved effect of PRP. In fact, several studies have reported that an excessive concentration of platelets may have inhibitory effects on cell proliferation or differentiation in populations such as tenocytes or adipose tissue-derived stem cells. Thus, the optimal platelet concentration for an optimized function is considered two- to threefold compared to blood levels [34, 35].

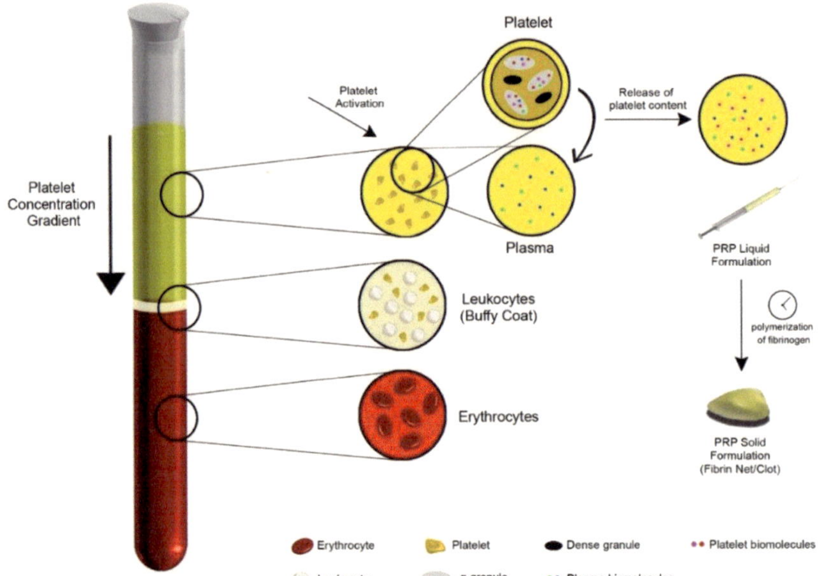

Figure 3.
Obtaining Platelet-Rich Plasma. After blood fractionation, the platelet-enriched plasma fraction is obtained. The activation of this fraction causes the release of the platelet content that together with the plasma molecules constitutes the effector biomolecules of the PRP. It also generates the polymerization of the fibrinogen that will create a network of fibrin where these biomolecules will be trapped, and that will be released progressively.

When separating the PRP from the rest of the blood fractions, there is the option to include or not the leukocyte layer, thus obtaining different PRP products, which will be detailed below. Although in some musculoskeletal disorders the use of Leukocyte-Rich PRP (LR-PRP) need further research, there is an increasingly broad consensus by which the use of leukocyte-poor PRP (LP-PRP) preparations is recommended for joint degeneration [36]. The inclusion of leukocytes in the PRP generated pro-inflammatory molecules that had negative effects on cell proliferation and chondrogenic differentiation as well as a worse regeneration of articular cartilage [37]. However, the fraction of red blood cells must be discarded in order to avoid the presence of erythrocytes in the PRP. The presence of erythrocytes in the PRP entails their own degradation processes such as hemolysis and eryptosis. As a result, products that promote inflammation and cellular stress are generated, which would hinder the beneficial action of PRP [38].

3.2.3 Platelet-Rich Plasma activation

The last step in the process to obtain PRP is the activation of platelets, through which its platelet content not only is released but also triggers the polymerization of fibrinogen in a fibrin mesh that traps the molecules. Thus, a controlled release system that delivers the molecules as it degrades is obtained. Activation can be exogenous either by physical methods such as freeze–thaw cycles or by the addition of certain substances (calcium chloride, thrombin). Some methods propose endogenous activation in which PRP is administered without prior activation and platelets are physiologically activated inside the body [39]. However, the use of exogenous activation allows a more versatile PRP, and depending on the time that has elapsed since the activation, different formulations are achieved at the point of care. The addition of calcium chloride as an activation method avoids the use of exogenous biological elements such as thrombin. It also prevents local hypocalcemia that can be caused by the calcium-chelating anticoagulants previously used in blood collection to prepare the PRP. Thus, PRP can be used as an injectable liquid formulation immediately after activation or as a fibrin membrane-clot minutes after adding the activator. In this case, and due to its consistency, this formulation can be used as a biological and autologous scaffold in surgical interventions that promote tissue repair [40].

3.3 Types of Platelet-Rich Plasma

As mentioned above, many variables may be involved in the obtaining process. It is not the intention of this chapter to delve into the large number of PRP types that exist both in the market and in the scientific literature. However, it is important to mention the variables that condition not only the type of PRP and therefore the different biological effects but also the classification systems (**Table 1**).

The three main variables that condition the obtaining of PRP, namely, number of platelets, presence or not of leukocytes, and activation, generate many different products under the PRP term which are necessary to differentiate. Not only a wide variety of products have emerged but also several classification systems that have attempted to clarify the inconsistency that accompanies the term PRP. Initially, the main difference was the presence or not of leukocytes. In the first classification of Dohan et al., PRPs could be distinguished in leukocyte-poor PRP and Leukocyte-Rich PRP, besides contemplating the fibrin presence [41]. Subsequently, Mishra [42] and DeLong [43] took into consideration the number of platelets and the activation of PRP. In the following classifications, the presence of erythrocytes [44] was also mentioned, and in recent years aspects such as recovery efficiency or centrifugation and application methods were addressed [45, 46], trying to classify as much as possible the different PRP products (**Table 1**).

As if that were not enough, new denominations are being coined in products derived from blood but that share the fundamental principles of PRP. This is the case of the Platelet-Rich Fibrin. These types appeared initially in the Dohan classification and refer to the fibrin clots that are formed either by centrifuging the blood without anticoagulants or by activating the liquid PRP and waiting for the formation of fibrin net, as mentioned above. A product derived from this is the hyperacute serum that is obtained with a procedure similar to that of the PRP but without using anticoagulants. Thus, after centrifugation of the blood, the upper fraction is a fibrin clot (Platelet-Rich Fibrin), which is squeezed to obtain the hyperacute serum [47]. It contains all the plasma and platelet biomolecules without coagulation proteins such as fibrinogen, namely, the product obtained is almost identical to the exudate gradually released from the fibrin net achieved after the activation of PRP. However, many growth factors present in the hyperacute serum will be eliminated quickly after its injection into the affected area due to its short half-life, whereas if they are released in a controlled manner as in the activated PRP, its time of action will be longer [48].

The lack of standardization is one of the main limitations in the application of PRP. Although all these products are called PRP, their composition may differ from many others and as a consequence their biological effects and clinical results. For instance, the presence of leukocytes determines the levels of pro-inflammatory molecules, and the activation or not of platelets affects the biomolecule release kinetics. Therefore, the comparison of PRP studies, assuming that it is the same product, yields contradictory data, so it is necessary to specify the type of PRP used in these works [49].

Variable type	Dohan [41]	Mishra [42]	PAW [43]	PLRA [44]	DEPA [45]	MARSPILL [46]
Composition	Leukocytes Fibrin	Platelets Leukocytes	Platelets Leukocytes Neutrophils	Platelets Leukocytes Neutrophils Erythrocytes	Platelets Leukocytes Erythrocytes	Platelets Leukocytes Erythrocytes
Activation	—	Activation	Activation	Activation	—	Activation Light
Others	—	—	—	—	Efficiency	Method Image guided Spin

Table 1.
Variables analyzed in the different classification systems.

4. Platelet-Rich Plasma and joint degeneration

4.1 Therapeutic potential of PRP in joint degeneration

As PRP is a product that contains a large number of bioactive molecules, it is wrong and impossible to define the effect of the PRP based on the isolated actions of each molecule. The biological effect of PRP depends not only on its molecules but also on its synergistic effect, which also considers interactions between molecules. Indeed, many PRP molecules are activated in the presence of others, or on the contrary many have antagonistic effects, conditioning the final effect of PRP.

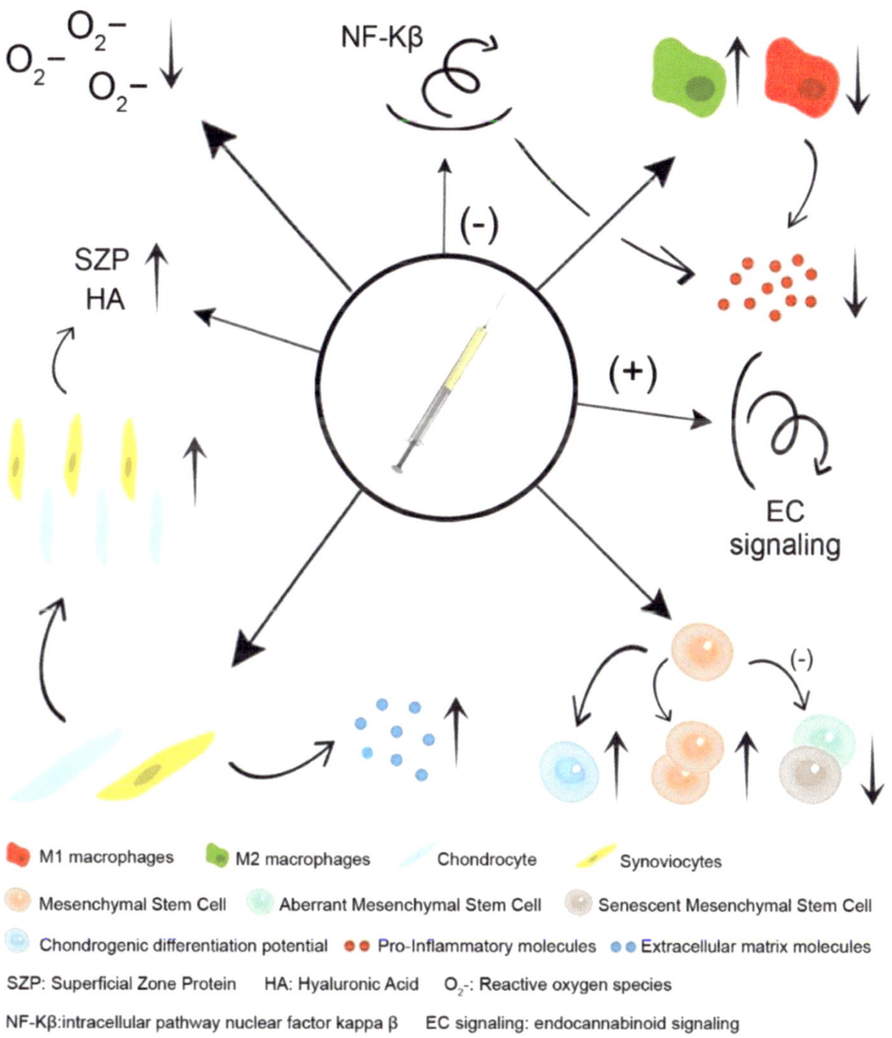

Figure 4.
Biological effects of Platelet-Rich Plasma on joint degeneration. The inhibition of the intracellular signaling pathway NF-Kβ, the reduction of reactive oxygen species, and the promotion of M2 macrophages cause the drop of pro-inflammatory molecule levels, achieving an anti-inflammatory effect. In addition, this decrease in pro-inflammatory molecules such as prostaglandin E2 achieves an analgesic effect, which is also favored by the activation of endocannabinoid systems. On the other hand, PRP modulates the cellular response, stimulating the proliferation of chondrocytes and synoviocytes, which increase the production of the substances responsible for lubrication. This modulation also affects mesenchymal stem cells, which increase their chondrogenic potential and decrease their aberrant and senescent forms.

Multiple actions are attributed to the PRP in the treatment of pathologies of the musculoskeletal system. However, this chapter will be limited to highlighting the effects that have the greatest impact on improving joint degeneration (**Figure 4**).

4.1.1 Anti-inflammatory effect

Due to the complex OA pathophysiology, inflammation can be both the cause and consequence of other pathological processes. Because of this, it is important to reverse the pro-inflammatory environment of this pathology and restore homeostasis of the joint to promote tissue repair. Many of the PRP molecules participate in the regulation of these inflammatory processes, which are key in the progression of the pathology. The anti-inflammatory effect of PRP is achieved through the action of its biomolecules at different levels. Molecules such as IGF-1 or HGF restore the original acquiescent state of cell populations from an inflammatory state because of joint degeneration. This effect occurs through the inhibition of the intracellular signaling pathway NF-Kβ by these molecules, and, as a result, the generation of pro-inflammatory molecules such as IL-β or TNF-α is reduced [50, 51]. The use of PRP rich in leukocytes can be especially important in this mechanism of action since, instead of inhibiting this inflammatory pathway, they activate it due to the presence of certain pro-inflammatory molecules in this type of PRP [37]. This inhibitory effect not only is limited to chondrocytes but also affects other cell populations such as fibroblast, osteoblasts [52], or macrophages [53]. The consequence of silencing this pathway in the different cell types of the joint is the drop in the inflammatory molecular levels of the synovial fluid, relieving the inflammatory environment [54].

Within its anti-inflammatory action, PRP also acts on macrophages by changing its phenotype. This effect may be indirect due to the decrease in pro-inflammatory molecules or direct by a direct action on the PRP components such as the microparticles produced by platelet apoptosis. The result is a phenotype shift of the macrophages from inflammatory (M1) to reparative (M2) phenotype, where the reduction of inflammation is favored and tissue repair is stimulated [55]. This effect is especially important in macrophages present in the synovial membrane. The increase in anti-inflammatory macrophages to the detriment of pro-inflammatories results in a decrease in inflammation of the synovial membrane, which is a hallmark of OA [56]. This polarization towards a reparative state may be due to the action of the interleukin 1 receptor antagonist, present in the PRP, which in addition to avoiding the inflammatory effect of IL-1 promotes the repair phenotype M2 of macrophages [57].

The inflammatory environment in the osteoarthritic joint is also potentiated by the increased presence of reactive oxygen species (ROS), which participate in the OA pathogenesis through synovium inflammation, cartilage degradation, or subchondral bone dysfunction [58]. PRP activates the antioxidant response element through the intracellular signaling pathway NrF2-ARE in osteoblasts [59]. This achieves an antioxidant and protective effect in these cell populations, avoiding damage caused by ROS increment.

The interaction of PRP biomolecules in the mechanisms that trigger inflammation results not only in a decrease in the levels of pro-inflammatory molecules and ROS but also in a promotion of gene expression related to anti-inflammatory action. It has recently been shown that gene expression of enzymes related to aggrecan destruction and metalloproteinase modulation, namely, metalloproteinase with thrombospondin motifs-5 (ADAMTS-5) and tissue inhibitor of metalloproteinases-1 (TIMP-1), are decreased in cartilage and synovium under the presence of PRP. However, gene expression related to the formation of collagen 1 and aggrecan is increased [60].

4.1.2 Analgesic effect

Pain is one of the most characteristic symptoms of OA and one of the most limiting factors for the patient, affecting its functionality and quality of life. One of the main causes of pain associated with joint degeneration is the inflammation that occurs. Solving the inflammatory problem would partly relieve the pain of the OA patient. This relief is one of the most observed effects in clinical studies since it is the most studied variable. However, it is necessary to deepen the mechanisms of action by which the PRP achieves the analgesic effect. During the inflammatory processes, molecules are generated by resident macrophages outstanding prostaglandin E_2 (PGE_2), which is one of the main causes of the inflammatory pain [61]. As mentioned earlier, PRP favors the change in macrophages from pro-inflammatory to anti-inflammatory phenotype as a consequence of the production of PGE2 and other pro-inflammatory molecule reductions [56]. In addition, the action of the PRP over the NF-Kβ pathway could also reduce the levels of substances that stimulate the nociceptors of the joint synovitis [62]. Therefore, inhibition of the synthesis of these substances is one of the mechanisms of action by which PRP reduces pain.

Although the action on inflammation may be the most predominant mechanism in pain relief, the implication of other pathways has been studied, namely, the peripheral endocannabinoid-mediated mechanism, which could be a promising therapeutic target in the synovial tissue of OA patients [63]. The influence of PRP on this signaling system is associated with the stimulation that occurs in the cells located in inflammatory environments. In the presence of PRR, these cells would generate analgesic substances such as anandamide and 2-arachidonoylglycerol, which are agonists of cannabinoid receptors 1 and 2. This effect is observed both in vitro and in vivo, with a lower nociceptive response in treated animals [62].

4.1.3 Biolubricanting effect

One of the problems associated with osteoarthritis is the lack of lubrication and therefore the increased friction in the joint. In a healthy joint, the synovial fluid has a natural lubricant function due to the presence of hyaluronic acid. The alteration of the components of the synovial fluid worsens the lubrication, deteriorating the cartilage. In addition, this layer of lubricant decreases progressively as the disease worsens, creating a vicious circle [64]. Restoring joint lubrication is one of the priorities to improve the course of the disease, and it is the purpose of intra-articular hyaluronic acid infiltrations [65].

The application of PRP also may restore joint lubrication through several mechanisms. First, it has a stimulating effect on the chondrocytes and synoviocytes, due to the fact that it not only enhances its proliferation but also increases the production of hyaluronic acid, improving the lubricating capacity of the synovial fluid [66–68]. Secondly, PRP also influences lubrication through the superficial zone protein (SZP) or lubricin. This protein synthesized by chondrocytes and synoviocytes acts as a chondroprotective barrier against direct contact in joints. PRP improves lubrication both directly, since it contains endogenous SZP, and indirectly by stimulating the SZP secretion by articular cartilage and synovium [69].

4.1.4 Cellular modulating effect

All the effects described above are generated through the interaction between growth factors and cell membrane receptors, triggering intracellular pathways and affecting gene expression that generates the biological effects. In addition to these, which are the most influential in the asymptomatic relief of OA, namely, inflammation, pain, and lubrication, there are other trophic and regulating effects that, although they do not have such a drastic clinical outcome, are necessary to promote tissue repair and reverse or slow down the disease.

PRP has demonstrated its biological effect over the chondrocytes of articular cartilage and its consequent impact on cartilage repair. Fice et al. published a systematic review including numerous in vitro and in vivo studies that showed the action of PRP on the cellular response [70]. On the one hand, it acts on cellular behavior, increasing growth, migration, and proliferation rates and reducing negative effects such as apoptosis. On the other hand, PRP enhances the synthesis of glycosaminoglycans (GAGs), proteoglycans, and collagen, improving the production of extracellular matrix.

In addition, stimulation of cartilage repair is also conditioned by the action of MSCs. They are able not only to differentiate into cells with specialized functions such as chondrocytes, osteoblasts, and adipocytes but also to release molecules and cellular signals that regulate the repair processes [71]. The behavior of MSCs in OA is modified, increasing in number in synovial fluid as the severity of the disease increases [72]. These MSCs come from resident joint niches such as the synovial membrane, the surface of the articular cartilage, and the subchondral bone, once again confirming the involvement of all the joint structures in the development of OA [17]. In this pathological environment, these cells have their function altered, losing their restorative activity [73]. Bearing this in mind, mesenchymal stem cells are considered a therapeutic target for the PRP to modulate its behavior and restore its physiological functions. Muiños-López et al. observed a decrease in MSCs in synovial fluid of patients with severe OA after the application of PRP directly into the subchondral bone [74]. The regulatory capacity of PRP on MSCs may be due to the direct action on their cellular response as well as the improvement of the biological environment in which the cells reside. Bone marrow-derived MSCs treated with PRP showed an increase in proliferation and chondrogenic capacity [75]. This increased proliferation was also observed in human adipose-derived stem cells, although their chondrogenic differentiation potential was retained [76]. Restoring tissue homeostasis where MSCs reside, for instance, by decreasing inflammation by inhibiting pro-inflammatory molecules, also improves the action of these cells. The attenuation of a TGF-β-mediated signaling excess in the subchondral bone during OA restores the dysfunction of the MSCs, preventing cartilage degeneration [77]. Liu et al. observed that intraosseous infiltrations of PRP promoted MSC cell proliferation and osteogenesis in an in vivo study, whereas adipogenesis, senescence, and oxidative stress were decreased [78].

4.2 Clinical translation

The transfer of the PRP from the laboratory to the clinical application has been very fast with extensive worldwide expansion. This has occurred in part because of its ease of obtaining and its high safety as an autologous product, and, as a consequence, more and more clinical studies are being published on the use of PRP in OA. It is not the intention of this chapter to analyze all these studies but to highlight the most relevant aspects of this translation. The latest published meta-analyses concluded that the use of intra-articular PRP infiltrations achieves effects on symptoms such as pain relief or improved function better than the use of hyaluronic acid or placebo especially for the long term [79–81]. Based on these data, it could be accepted that the PRP has evolved from being a promising alternative to a real option for clinicians and patients.

However, it should not be forgotten that it is necessary to continue to carry out high-quality clinical studies to clarify possible doubts and achieve the ideal protocol for both obtaining and applying PRP products [82]. Some of the clinical studies carried out have attempted to elucidate this type of questions, the presence of leukocytes being one of the most critical issues. Several authors have studied the clinical effect of including leukocytes in the PRP. Mariani et al. studied the pro-inflammatory effect that intra-articular infiltrations of Leukocyte-Rich PRP could have. Surprisingly, and contrary to the in vitro studies, patients who received this treatment did not experience an increase of pro-inflammatory molecules in the synovial fluid or plasma in the short or long term [83]. These data were confirmed in a meta-analysis where there were no differences in adverse reactions between PRP with and without leukocytes, being very rare and local such as pain and inflammation. However, as far as efficacy is concerned, this same work carried out by Riboh et al. showed that PRP poor in leukocytes had significantly better results than those obtained by hyaluronic acid and placebo, whereas this difference did not occur in PRP rich in leukocytes. Therefore, according to the studies carried out in this matter, the inclusion of leukocytes in the PRP does not affect the safety of the product but does diminish its effectiveness in the treatment of knee OA [36]. In spite of these advances, it is necessary to continue studying the rest of the composition variables that may condition the clinical response of the PRP, such as platelet concentration. Recent studies suggest that a concentration below fivefold blood platelet concentration is recommended [84].

Not only the variables related to the obtaining or composition of the PRP products condition the clinical effect of this therapy but also the different methods of application. Several clinical studies addressed the effect of a single or repeated administration of intra-articular infiltrations of PRP. A first group of studies focused on analyzing the differences between a single infiltration of PRP and several repeated infiltrations every 1 or 2 weeks. These studies demonstrated that PRP obtained better results than control treatment and, in addition, patients who received repeated intra-articular infiltrations of PRP achieved better clinical response on items such as pain, symptomatology, and function [85–87]. Other studies analyzed the effect of applying several cycles of PRP infiltrations, referring to a cycle as a series of repeated infiltrations in a short period of time. Gobbi et al. compared the efficacy of administration of one PRP cycle against two PRP cycles separated by 1 year, one cycle being three intra-articular infiltrations of PRP in 1 month. In both groups, there was an improvement in patients 1 year after the first cycle, which was accentuated at 18 months after the application of a second cycle [88]. Vaquerizo et al. conducted a similar study comparing patients treated with one PRP cycle with patients treated with two PRP cycles separated by 6 months, one cycle being three weekly intra-articular PRP infiltrations. The results showed that although there were no significant differences in pain improvement, patients who received two cycles had better symptoms and functionality 1 year after treatment [89]. Thus, the different studies that analyze this variable recommend the application of repeated PRP injections instead of isolated ones.

Following with the PRP administration modality, it is important to remember that the mechanism of action of PRP biomolecules is cell stimulation and improvement of the biological environment to favor tissue repair. Furthermore, as explained at the beginning of this chapter, OA is an alteration of the whole joint and not just a few elements. Considering these two assumptions, it would be advisable to act on the majority of the tissues involved in the joint and especially on those that perform a more predominant biological function. When PRP is intra-articularly administered, it soaked the articular space, reaching and acting on the cells present both in the synovial membrane and on the articular surface. However, this route of administration does not reach the subchondral bone which communicates with the cartilage, especially in OA case, and it is fundamental both in the maintenance

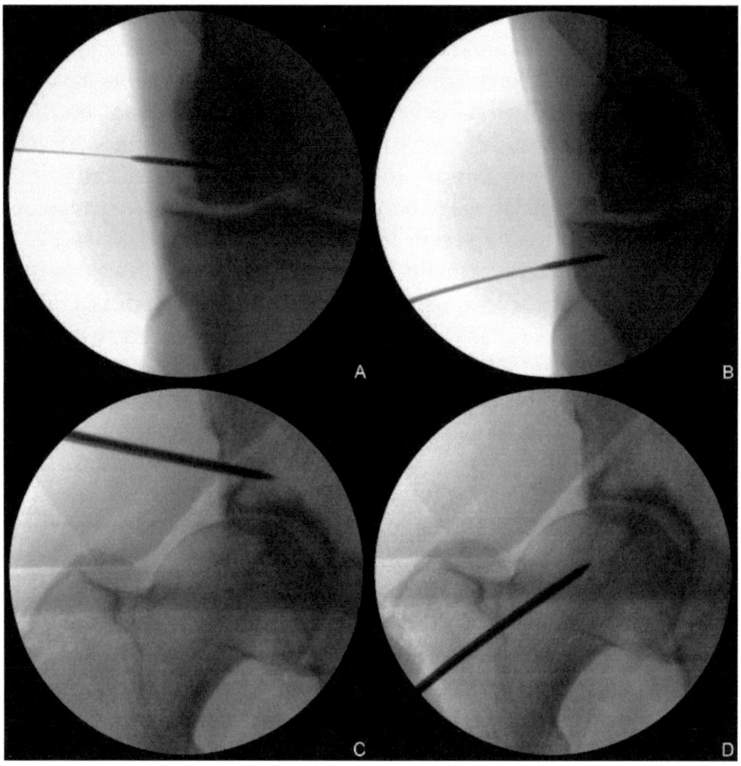

Figure 5.
Intraosseous administration of PRP. Intraosseous PRP administrations allow the subchondral bone to be reached and its therapeutic effect to be extended. Intraosseous infiltrations are applied in the femoral condyle (A) and tibial plateau (B) in patients with knee OA and in the acetabulum (C) and femoral head (D) in cases of hip OA.

of homeostasis and in the pathophysiology of joint degeneration [17]. In order to extend the range of action of the PRP and also act on the subchondral bone, Sánchez et al. described the technique of PRP intraosseous infiltrations (**Figure 5**). This method of application combines conventional intra-articular injection of PRP with intraosseous infiltrations into the subchondral bone of the femoral condyle and tibial plateau in severe cases of knee OA [90]. Afterward, this technique was adapted to treat advanced cases of hip OA, combining intra-articular infiltration with intraosseous infiltrations into the femoral head and acetabulum [91]. In both cases, intraosseous administration must be assisted by imaging, ultrasound, or fluoroscopy, to ensure correct delivery in the required area.

The first published works carried out using this technique provided promising results. In a pilot study performed with patients who presented knee OA of grades 3 and 4 according to the Ahlbäck scale, pain was significantly reduced, and an increase in joint function was observed at 6 months after receiving the combination of intra-articular and intraosseous PRP injections. In addition, the number of MSCs present in the synovial fluid decreased after this treatment [92]. This finding was not observed in patients treated only with intra-articular infiltrations, suggesting the importance of the subchondral bone in the modulation of cellular response in joint degeneration [74]. Following the same trend, an observational study compared the intra-articular administration of PRP versus the combination of intra-articular and intraosseous injections in patients with severe knee OA. The results of this study showed that although there was no difference between both groups at 2 months after treatment, patients who received the PRP intraosseously showed clinically superior results at 6 and 12 months [93]. Su et al. conducted a clinical trial in which, in addition to comparing intra-articular against intraosseous injections, they used hyaluronic acid as a control treatment. The patients enrolled in this study presented knee OA of grades 2 and 3 according to the Kellgren-Lawrence scale. The results achieved with treatment based on intraosseous infiltrations of PRP were superior to those obtained with both intra-articular PRP and hyaluronic acid [94]. No severe adverse effects were reported in any of these studies, and they were limited to pain after infiltrations. One of the characteristics of the subchondral bone in patients with knee OA is the presence of fibroneurovascular proliferation. Although the PRP contains proangiogenic and profibrotic molecules, no basic or clinical study showed the uncontrolled induction of this effect after the application of intraosseous PRP [22].

Finally, intra-articular injections of MSCs derived from various sources associated with PRP were analyzed in some studies. The vehiculization of MSCs in PRP could entail an improvement in cell viability and may be translated into better clinical results. Although studies performed with both bone marrow [95, 96]- and stroma fraction [97, 98]-derived MSCs showed improvement in these patients after the application of this therapeutic combination, the association of PRP with the MSCs did not lead to a greater clinical improvement in patients. However, the therapeutic potential of the synergy of both therapies justifies further research in this field.

5. Conclusions

Joint degeneration is a pathology that affects a large part of the population, deteriorating their quality of life being disabling in many cases. It is also related to aging and unhealthy lifestyle habits; thus it is expected that its prevalence will increase in the coming years, assuming a great cost to health systems. Current conventional treatments focus on symptomatic relief without addressing the cause of the disease. Because of this, new treatments based on regenerative medicine are emerging in order to expand the therapeutic arsenal and delay or prevent joint replacement, which is currently the only definitive solution for patients. Moreover, in order to achieve an optimal treatment for joint degeneration, it must be understood that the joint works as a whole organ. All elements of the joint participate in the maintenance of homeostasis, the synovial membrane, cartilage, and subchondral bone being key for biological balance.

This balance could be maintained or restored by means of several biological therapies such as PRP that is a cocktail of plasma and platelet biomolecules, and it is obtained after fractionating small blood volumes by centrifugation. PRP has a great versatility since it allows its use through different types of formulations, being able to be applied both in outpatient infiltrations and surgical interventions. The therapeutic potential of PRP in joint degeneration lies in its ability to modulate inflammation, lubrication, and pain, acting on different cell populations to create a biological environment conducive to tissue repair. However, the variety in the composition of PRP products leads to different biological effects and consequently contradictory clinical results. It is, therefore, necessary to identify and characterize the PRP used in order to advance both research and clinical practice.

The success of the PRP also depends on the method of clinical application. The administration of PRP has to cover the main joint tissues so that the biological effects of PRP act over the cells of in order to reverse the course of the pathology. Although the safety and ease of obtaining PRP have allowed a quick transfer from the laboratory to the hospital, much is still unknown about this therapy, and further basic and clinical research is needed.

Author details

Mikel Sánchez[1,2]*, Maider Beitia[2], Orlando Pompei[1], Cristina Jorquera[2], Pello Sánchez[2], Jorge Knörr[1], Francisco Soldado[1], Leonor López[1], Jaime Oraa[1], Ane Miren Bilbao[1], Nicolás Fiz[1], Jorge Guadilla[1], Beatriz Aizpurua[1], Juan Azofra[1] and Diego Delgado[2]

1 Arthroscopic Surgery Unit, Hospital Vithas San José, Vitoria-Gasteiz, Spain

2 Advanced Biological Therapy Unit, Hospital Vithas San José, Vitoria-Gasteiz, Spain

*Address all correspondence to: mikel.sanchez@ucatrauma.com

References

[1] O'Neill TW, McCabe PS, McBeth J. Update on the epidemiology, risk factors and disease outcomes of osteoarthritis. Best Practice & Research. Clinical Rheumatology. 2018;**32**(2):312-326. DOI: 10.1016/j.berh.2018.10.007

[2] Berenbaum F. Osteoarthritis as an inflammatory disease (osteoarthritis is not osteoarthrosis!). Osteoarthritis and Cartilage. 2013;**21**(1):16-21. DOI: 10.1016/j.joca.2012.11.012

[3] Lohmander LS, Roos EM. Clinical update: Treating osteoarthritis. Lancet. 2007;**370**(9605):2082-2084. DOI: 10.1016/S0140-6736(07)61879-0

[4] Lum ZC, Shieh AK, Dorr LD. Why total knees fail-a modern perspective review. World Journal of Orthopedics. 2018;**9**(4):60-64. DOI: 10.5312/wjo.v9.i4.60

[5] Chen A, Gupte C, Akhtar K, Smith P, Cobb J. The global economic cost of osteoarthritis: How the UK compares. Art. 2012;**2012**:698709. DOI: 10.1155/2012/698709

[6] Andia I, Maffulli N. New biotechnologies for musculoskeletal injuries. The Surgeon. 2019;**17**(4):244-255. DOI: 10.1016/j.surge.2018.08.004

[7] O'Connell B, Wragg NM, Wilson SL.The use of PRP injections in the management of knee osteoarthritis. Cell and Tissue Research. 2019;**376**(2):143-152. DOI: 10.1007/s00441-019-02996-x

[8] Loeser RF, Goldring SR, Scanzello CR, Goldring MB. Osteoarthritis: A disease of the joint as an organ. Arthritis and Rheumatism. 2012;**64**(6):1697-1707. DOI: 10.1002/art.34453

[9] Buchman TG. The community of the self. Nature. 2002;**420**(6912):246-251. DOI: 10.1038/nature01260

[10] Kjaer M. Role of extracellular matrix in adaptation of tendon and skeletal muscle to mechanical loading. Physiological Reviews. 2004;**84**(2):649-698. DOI: 10.1152/physrev.00031.2003

[11] Brandt KD, Radin EL, Dieppe PA, van de Putte L. Yet more evidence that osteoarthritis is not a cartilage disease. Annals of the Rheumatic Diseases. 2006;**65**(10):1261-1264. DOI: 10.1136/ard.2006.058347

[12] Hoffmann A, Gross G. Tendon and ligament engineering in the adult organism: Mesenchymal stem cells and gene-therapeutic approaches. International Orthopaedics. 2007;**31**(6):791-797. DOI: 10.1007/s00264-007-0395-9

[13] Fox AJ, Wanivenhaus F, Burge AJ, Warren RF, Rodeo SA. The human meniscus: A review of anatomy, function, injury, and advances in treatment. Clinical Anatomy. 2015;**28**(2):269-287. DOI: 10.1002/ca.22456

[14] de Sousa EB, Casado PL, Moura Neto V, Duarte ME, Aguiar DP. Synovial fluid and synovial membrane mesenchymal stem cells: Latest discoveries and therapeutic perspectives. Stem Cell Research & Therapy. 2014;**5**(5):112. DOI: 10.1186/scrt501

[15] Smith MD. The normal synovium. The Open Rheumatology Journal. 2011;**5**:100-106. DOI: 10.2174/1874312901105010100

[16] Anitua E, Sánchez M, Orive G, Padilla S. A biological therapy to osteoarthritis treatment using platelet-rich plasma. Expert Opinion on Biological Therapy. 2013;**13**(8):1161-1172. DOI: 10.1517/14712598.2013.801450

[17] Sánchez M, Anitua E, Delgado D, Sanchez P, Prado R, Goiriena JJ, et al. A new strategy to tackle severe knee osteoarthritis: Combination of intra-articular and intraosseous injections of platelet rich plasma. Expert Opinion on Biological Therapy. 2016;**16**(5):627-643. DOI: 10.1517/14712598.2016.1157162

[18] Tchetina EV. Developmental mechanisms in articular cartilage degradation in osteoarthritis. Art. 2011;**2011**:683970. DOI: 10.1155/2011/683970

[19] Goldring MB, Marcu KB. Cartilage homeostasis in health and rheumatic diseases. Arthritis Research & Therapy. 2009;**11**(3):224. DOI: 10.1186/ar2592

[20] Nam J, Aguda BD, Rath B, Agarwal S. Biomechanical thresholds regulate inflammation through the NF-kappaB pathway: Experiments and modeling. PLoS One. 2009;**4**(4):e5262. DOI: 10.1371/journal.pone.0005262

[21] Scanzello CR, Goldring SR. The role of synovitis in osteoarthritis pathogenesis. Bone. 2012;**51**(2):249-257. DOI: 10.1016/j.bone.2012.02.012

[22] Delgado D, Garate A, Vincent H, Bilbao AM, Patel R, Fiz N, et al. Current concepts in intraosseous platelet-rich plasma injections for knee osteoarthritis. Journal of Clinical Orthopaedics and Trauma. 2019;**10**(1):36-41. DOI: 10.1016/j.jcot.2018.09.017

[23] Krasnokutsky S, Belitskaya-Lévy I, Bencardino J, Samuels J, Attur M, Regatte R, et al. Quantitative magnetic resonance imaging evidence of synovial proliferation is associated with radiographic severity of knee osteoarthritis. Arthritis and Rheumatism. 2011;**63**(10):2983-2991. DOI: 10.1002/art.30471

[24] Suri S, Walsh DA. Osteochondral alterations in osteoarthritis. Bone. 2012;**51**(2):204-211. DOI: 10.1016/j.bone.2011.10.010

[25] Katsuragawa Y, Saitoh K, Tanaka N, Wake M, Ikeda Y, Furukawa H, et al. Changes of human menisci in osteoarthritic knee joints. Osteoarthritis and Cartilage. 2010;**18**(9):1133-1143. DOI: 10.1016/j.joca.2010.05.017

[26] Hasegawa A, Otsuki S, Pauli C, Miyaki S, Patil S, Steklov N, et al. Anterior cruciate ligament changes in the human knee joint in aging and osteoarthritis. Arthritis and Rheumatism. 2012;**64**(3):696-704. DOI: 10.1002/art.33417

[27] Shorter E, Sannicandro AJ, Poulet B, Goljanek-Whysall K. Skeletal muscle wasting and its relationship with osteoarthritis: A mini-review of mechanisms and current interventions. Current Rheumatology Reports. 2019;**21**(8):40. DOI: 10.1007/s11926-019-0839-4

[28] Machlus KR, Italiano JE Jr. The incredible journey: From megakaryocyte development to platelet formation. The Journal of Cell Biology. 2013;**201**(6):785-796. DOI: 10.1083/jcb.201304054

[29] Gremmel T, Frelinger AL 3rd, Michelson AD. Platelet physiology. Seminars in Thrombosis and Hemostasis. 2016;**42**(3):191-204. DOI: 10.1055/s-0035-1564835

[30] De Paoli SH, Tegegn TZ, Elhelu OK, Strader MB, Patel M, Diduch LL, et al. Dissecting the biochemical architecture and morphological release pathways of the human platelet extracellular vesiculome. Cellular and Molecular Life Sciences. 2018;**75**(20):3781-3801. DOI: 10.1007/s00018-018-2771-6

[31] Padilla S, Sánchez M, Orive G, Anitua E. Human-based biological and biomimetic autologous therapies for musculoskeletal tissue

regeneration. Trends in Biotechnology. 2017;**35**(3):192-202

[32] Spezia J, Hermann PB, Comar SR, Picheth G, Henneberg R, Utiyama SRR. Anticoagulant choices affect the mean platelet volume measurement by impedance. Clinical Laboratory. 2018;**64**:217-220. DOI: 10.7754/Clin.Lab.2017.170806

[33] Wisgrill L, Lamm C, Hartmann J, Preißing F, Dragosits K, Bee A, et al. Peripheral blood microvesicles secretion is influenced by storage time, temperature, and anticoagulants. Cytometry. Part A. 2016;**89**(7):663-672. DOI: 10.1002/cyto.a.22892

[34] Giusti I, D'Ascenzo S, Mancò A, Di Stefano G, Di Francesco M, Rughetti A, et al. Platelet concentration in platelet-rich plasma affects tenocyte behavior in vitro. BioMed Research International. 2014;**2014**:630870. DOI: 10.1155/2014/630870

[35] Felthaus O, Prantl L, Skaff-Schwarze M, Klein S, Anker A, Ranieri M, et al. Assessing clinical implications and perspectives of the pathophysiological effects of erythrocytes and plasma free hemoglobin in autologous biologics for use in musculoskeletal regenerative medicine therapies. A review. Regenerative Therapy. 2019;**11**:56-64. DOI: 10.1016/j.reth.2019.03.009

[36] Riboh JC, Saltzman BM, Yanke AB, Fortier L, Cole BJ. Effect of leukocyte concentration on the efficacy of platelet-rich plasma in the treatment of knee osteoarthritis. The American Journal of Sports Medicine. 2016;**44**(3):792-800. DOI: 10.1177/0363546515580787

[37] Xu Z, Yin W, Zhang Y, Qi X, Chen Y, Xie X, et al. Comparative evaluation of leukocyte- and platelet-rich plasma and pure platelet-rich plasma for cartilage regeneration. Scientific Reports. 2017;**7**:43301. DOI: 10.1038/srep43301

[38] Everts PA, Malanga GA, Paul RV, Rothenberg J, Stephens N, Mautner KR. Assessing clinical implications and perspectives of the pathophysiological effects of erythrocytes and plasma free hemoglobin in autologous biologics for use in musculoskeletal regenerative medicine therapies. A review. Regenerative Therapy. 2019;**11**:56-64. DOI: 10.1016/j.reth.2019.03.009

[39] Kikuchi N, Yoshioka T, Taniguchi Y, Sugaya H, Arai N, Kanamori A, et al. Optimization of leukocyte-poor platelet-rich plasma preparation: A validation study of leukocyte-poor platelet-rich plasma obtained using different preparer, storage, and activation methods. Journal of Experimental Orthopaedics. 2019;**6**(1):24. DOI: 10.1186/s40634-019-0190-8

[40] Anitua E, Nurden P, Prado R, Nurden AT, Padilla S. Autologous fibrin scaffolds: When platelet- and plasma-derived biomolecules meet fibrin. Biomaterials. 2019;**192**:440-460. DOI: 10.1016/j.biomaterials.2018.11.029

[41] Dohan Ehrenfest DM, Rasmusson L, Albrektsson T. Classification of platelet concentrates: From pure platelet-rich plasma (P-PRP) to leucocyte- and platelet-rich fibrin (L-PRF). Trends in Biotechnology. 2009;**27**(3):158-167. DOI: 10.1016/j.tibtech.2008.11.009

[42] Mishra A, Harmon K, Woodall J, Vieira A. Sports medicine applications of platelet rich plasma. Current Pharmaceutical Biotechnology. 2012;**13**(7):1185-1195. DOI: 10.2174/138920112800624283

[43] DeLong JM, Russell RP, Mazzocca AD. Platelet-rich plasma: The PAW classification system. Arthroscopy. 2012;**28**(7):998-1009. DOI: 10.1016/j.arthro.2012.04.148

[44] Mautner K, Malanga GA, Smith J, Shiple B, Ibrahim V, Sampson S, et al.

A call for a standard classification system for future biologic research: The rationale for new PRP nomenclature. PM&R: The Journal of Injury, Function, and Rehabilitation. 2015;**7**(4 Suppl):S53-S59. DOI: 10.1016/j.pmrj.2015.02.005

[45] Magalon J, Chateau AL, Bertrand B, Louis ML, Silvestre A, Giraudo L, et al. DEPA classification: A proposal for standardising PRP use and a retrospective application of available devices. BMJ Open Sport & Exercise Medicine. 2016;**2**(1):e000060. DOI: 10.1136/bmjsem-2015-000060

[46] Lana JFSD, Purita J, Paulus C, Huber SC, Rodrigues BL, Rodrigues AA, et al. Contributions for classification of platelet rich plasma - proposal of a new classification: MARSPILL. Regenerative Medicine. 2017;**12**(5):565-574. DOI: 10.2217/rme-2017-0042

[47] Kardos D, Simon M, Vácz G, Hinsenkamp A, Holczer T, Cseh D, et al. The composition of hyperacute serum and platelet-rich plasma is markedly different despite the similar production method. International Journal of Molecular Sciences. 2019;**20**(3):E721. DOI: 10.3390/ijms20030721

[48] Anitua E, Zalduendo MM, Alkhraisat MH, Orive G. Release kinetics of platelet-derived and plasma-derived growth factors from autologous plasma rich in growth factors. Annals of Anatomy. 2013;**195**(5):461-466. DOI: 10.1016/j.aanat.2013.04.004

[49] Rossi LA, Murray IR, Chu CR, Muschler GF, Rodeo SA, Piuzzi NS. Classification systems for platelet-rich plasma. The Bone & Joint Journal. 2019;**101-B**(8):891-896. DOI: 10.1302/0301-620X.101B8.BJJ-2019-0037.R1

[50] Bendinelli P, Matteucci E, Dogliotti G, Corsi MM, Banfi G, Maroni P, et al. Molecular basis of anti-inflammatory action of platelet-rich plasma on human chondrocytes: Mechanisms of NF-κB inhibition via HGF. Journal of Cellular Physiology. 2010;**225**(3):757-766. DOI: 10.1002/jcp.22274

[51] van Buul GM, Koevoet WL, Kops N, Bos PK, Verhaar JA, Weinans H, et al. Platelet-rich plasma releasate inhibits inflammatory processes in osteoarthritic chondrocytes. The American Journal of Sports Medicine. 2011;**39**(11):2362-2370. DOI: 10.1177/0363546511419278

[52] Anitua E, Zalduendo M, Troya M, Padilla S, Orive G. Leukocyte inclusion within a platelet rich plasma-derived fibrin scaffold stimulates a more pro-inflammatory environment and alters fibrin properties. PLoS One. 2015;**10**(3):e0121713. DOI: 10.1371/journal.pone.0121713

[53] Coudriet GM, He J, Trucco M, Mars WM, Piganelli JD. Hepatocyte growth factor modulates interleukin-6 production in bone marrow derived macrophages: Implications for inflammatory mediated diseases. PLoS One. 2010;**5**(11):e15384. DOI: 10.1371/journal.pone.0015384

[54] Huang G, Hua S, Yang T, Ma J, Yu W, Chen X. Platelet-rich plasma shows beneficial effects for patients with knee osteoarthritis by suppressing inflammatory factors. Experimental and Therapeutic Medicine. 2018;**15**(3):3096-3102. DOI: 10.3892/etm.2018.5794

[55] Vasina EM, Cauwenberghs S, Feijge MAH, Heemskerk JWM, Weber C, Koenen RR. Microparticles from apoptotic platelets promote resident macrophage differentiation. Cell Death & Disease. 2011;**2**(11):e233. DOI: 10.1038/cddis.2011.115

[56] Khatab S, van Buul GM, Kops N, Bastiaansen-Jenniskens YM, Bos PK, Verhaar JA, et al. Intra-articular injections of platelet-rich plasma

Releasate reduce pain and synovial inflammation in a mouse model of osteoarthritis. The American Journal of Sports Medicine. 2018;**46**(4):977-986. DOI: 10.1177/0363546517750635

[57] Lepetsos P, Papavassiliou AG. ROS/oxidative stress signaling in osteoarthritis. Biochimica et Biophysica Acta. 2016;**1862**(4):576-591. DOI: 10.1016/j.bbadis.2016.01.003

[58] Luz-Crawford P, Djouad F, Toupet K, Bony C, Franquesa M, Hoogduijn MJ, et al. Mesenchymal stem cell-derived interleukin 1 receptor antagonist promotes macrophage polarization and inhibits B cell differentiation. Stem Cells. 2016;**34**(2):483-492. DOI: 10.1002/stem.2254

[59] Tohidnezhad M, Wruck CJ, Slowik A, Kweider N, Beckmann R, Bayer A, et al. Role of platelet-released growth factors in detoxification of reactive oxygen species in osteoblasts. Bone. 2014;**65**:9-17. DOI: 10.1016/j.bone.2014.04.029

[60] O'Brien D, Kia C, Beebe R, Macken C, Bell R, Cote M, et al. Evaluating the effects of platelet-rich plasma and amniotic viscous fluid on inflammatory markers in a human coculture model for osteoarthritis. Arthroscopy. 2019;**35**(8):2421-2433. DOI: 10.1016/j.arthro.2019.03.021

[61] Ulmann L, Hirbec H, Rassendren F. P2X4 receptors mediate PGE2 release by tissue-resident macrophages and initiate inflammatory pain. The EMBO Journal. 2010;**29**(14):2290-2300. DOI: 10.1038/emboj.2010

[62] Descalzi F, Ulivi V, Cancedda R, Piscitelli F, Luongo L, Guida F, et al. Platelet-richplasmaexertsantinociceptive activity by a peripheral endocannabinoid-related mechanism. Tissue Engineering. Part A. 2013;**19**(19-20):2120-2129. DOI: 10.1089/ten.TEA.2012.0557

[63] Richardson D, Pearson RG, Kurian N, Latif ML, Garle MJ, Barrett DA, et al. Characterisation of the cannabinoid receptor system in synovial tissue and fluid in patients with osteoarthritis and rheumatoid arthritis. Arthritis Research & Therapy. 2008;**10**(2):R43. DOI: 10.1186/ar2401

[64] Corvelli M, Che B, Saeui C, Singh A, Elisseeff J. Biodynamic performance of hyaluronic acid versus synovial fluid of the knee in osteoarthritis. Methods. 2015;**84**:90-98. DOI: 10.1016/j.ymeth.2015.03.019

[65] Nicholls M, Manjoo A, Shaw P, Niazi F, Rosen J. A comparison between rheological properties of intra-articular hyaluronic acid preparations and reported human synovial fluid. Advances in Therapy. 2018;**35**(4):523-530. DOI: 10.1007/s12325-018-0688-y

[66] Anitua E, Sanchez M, De la Fuente M, Zalduendo MM, Orive G. Plasma rich in growth factors (PRGF-Endoret) stimulates tendon and synovial fibroblasts migration and improves the biological properties of hyaluronic acid. Knee Surgery, Sports Traumatology, Arthroscopy. 2012;**20**(9):1657-1665. DOI: 10.1007/s00167-011-1697-4

[67] Cavallo C, Filardo G, Mariani E, Kon E, Marcacci M, Pereira Ruiz MT, et al. Comparison of platelet-rich plasma formulations for cartilage healing: An in vitro study. The Journal of Bone and Joint Surgery. American Volume. 2014;**96**(5):423-429. DOI: 10.2106/JBJS.M.00726

[68] Gilbertie JM, Long JM, Schubert AG, Berglund AK, Schaer TP, Schnabel LV. Pooled platelet-rich plasma lysate therapy increases synoviocyte proliferation and hyaluronic acid production while protecting chondrocytes from synoviocyte-derived inflammatory mediators. Frontiers in Veterinary Science. 2018;**5**:150. DOI: 10.3389/fvets.2018.00150

[69] Sakata R, McNary SM, Miyatake K, Lee CA, Van den Bogaerde JM, Marder RA, et al. Stimulation of the superficial zone protein and lubrication in the articular cartilage by human platelet-rich plasma. The American Journal of Sports Medicine. 2015;**43**(6):1467-1473. DOI: 10.1177/0363546515575023

[70] Fice MP, Miller JC, Christian R, Hannon CP, Smyth N, Murawski CD, et al. The role of platelet-rich plasma in cartilage pathology: An updated systematic review of the basic science evidence. Arthroscopy. 2019;**35**(3):961-976.e3. DOI: 10.1016/j.arthro.2018.10.125

[71] Caplan AI. Adult mesenchymal stem cells: When, where, and how. Stem Cells International. 2015;**2015**:628767. DOI: 10.1155/2015/628767

[72] Sekiya I, Ojima M, Suzuki S, Yamaga M, Horie M, Koga H, et al. Human mesenchymal stem cells in synovial fluid increase in the knee with degenerated cartilage and osteoarthritis. Journal of Orthopaedic Research. 2012;**30**(6):943-949. DOI: 10.1002/jor.22029

[73] Campbell TM, Churchman SM, Gomez A, McGonagle D, Conaghan PG, Ponchel F, et al. Mesenchymal stem cell alterations in bone marrow lesions in patients with hip osteoarthritis. Arthritis & Rhematology. 2016;**68**(7):1648-1659. DOI: 10.1002/art.39622

[74] Muiños-López E, Delgado D, Sánchez P, Paiva B, Anitua E, Fiz N, et al. Modulation of synovial fluid-derived mesenchymal stem cells by intra-articular and intraosseous platelet rich plasma administration. Stem Cells International. 2016;**2016**:1247950. DOI: 10.1155/2016/1247950

[75] Krüger JP, Hondke S, Endres M, Pruss A, Siclari A, Kaps C. Human platelet-rich plasma stimulates migration and chondrogenic differentiation of human subchondral progenitor cells. Journal of Orthopaedic Research. 2012;**30**(6):845-852. DOI: 10.1002/jor.22005

[76] Hildner F, Eder MJ, Hofer K, Aberl J, Redl H, van Griensven M, et al. Human platelet lysate successfully promotes proliferation and subsequent chondrogenic differentiation of adipose-derived stem cells: A comparison with articular chondrocytes. Journal of Tissue Engineering and Regenerative Medicine. 2015;**9**(7):808-818. DOI: 10.1002/term

[77] Zhen G, Wen C, Jia X, Li Y, Crane JL, Mears SC, et al. Inhibition of TGF-β signaling in mesenchymal stem cells of subchondral bone attenuates osteoarthritis. Nature Medicine. 2013;**19**(6):704-712. DOI: 10.1038/nm.3143

[78] Liu HY, Huang CF, Lin TC, Tsai CY, Tina Chen SY, Liu A, et al. Delayed animal aging through the recovery of stem cell senescence by platelet rich plasma. Biomaterials. 2014;**35**(37):9767-9776. DOI: 10.1016/j.biomaterials.2014.08.034

[79] Han Y, Huang H, Pan J, Lin J, Zeng L, Liang G, et al. Meta-analysis comparing platelet-rich plasma vs hyaluronic acid injection in patients with knee osteoarthritis. Pain Medicine. 2019;**20**(7):1418-1429. DOI: 10.1093/pm/pnz011

[80] Dai WL, Zhou AG, Zhang H, Zhang J. Efficacy of platelet-rich plasma in the treatment of knee osteoarthritis: A meta-analysis of randomized controlled trials. Arthroscopy. 2017;**33**(3):659-670.e1. DOI: 10.1016/j.arthro.2016.09.024

[81] Xing D, Wang B, Zhang W, Yang Z, Hou Y, Chen Y, et al. Intra-articular platelet-rich plasma injections for knee osteoarthritis: An overview of

systematic reviews and risk of bias considerations. International Journal of Rheumatic Diseases. 2017;**20**(11):1612-1630. DOI: 10.1111/1756-185X.13233

[82] Zhang HF, Wang CG, Li H, Huang YT, Li ZJ. Intra-articular platelet-rich plasma versus hyaluronic acid in the treatment of knee osteoarthritis: A meta-analysis. Drug Design, Development and Therapy. 2018;**12**:445-453. DOI: 10.2147/DDDT.S156724

[83] Mariani E, Canella V, Cattini L, Kon E, Marcacci M, Di Matteo B, et al. Leukocyte-rich platelet-rich plasma injections do not up-modulate intra-articular pro-inflammatory cytokines in the osteoarthritic knee. PLoS One. 2016;**11**(6):e0156137. DOI: 10.1371/journal.pone.0156137

[84] Milants C, Bruyère O, Kaux JF. Responders to platelet-rich plasma in osteoarthritis: A technical analysis. BioMed Research International. 2017;**2017**:7538604. DOI: 10.1155/2017/7538604

[85] Tavassoli M, Janmohammadi N, Hosseini A, Khafri S, Esmaeilnejad-Ganji SM. Single- and double-dose of platelet-rich plasma versus hyaluronic acid for treatment of knee osteoarthritis: A randomized controlled trial. World Journal of Orthopedics. 2019;**10**(9):310-326. DOI: 10.5312/wjo.v10.i9.310

[86] Görmeli G, Görmeli CA, Ataoglu B, Çolak C, Aslantürk O, Ertem K. Multiple PRP injections are more effective than single injections and hyaluronic acid in knees with early osteoarthritis: A randomized, double-blind, placebo-controlled trial. Knee Surgery, Sports Traumatology, Arthroscopy. 2017;**25**(3):958-965. DOI: 10.1007/s00167-015-3705-6

[87] Kavadar G, Demircioglu DT, Celik MY, Emre TY. Effectiveness of platelet-rich plasma in the treatment of moderate knee osteoarthritis: A randomized prospective study. Journal of Physical Therapy Science. 2015;**27**(12):3863-3867. DOI: 10.1589/jpts.27.3863

[88] Gobbi A, Lad D, Karnatzikos G. The effects of repeated intra-articular PRP injections on clinical outcomes of early osteoarthritis of the knee. Knee Surgery, Sports Traumatology, Arthroscopy. 2015;**23**(8):2170-2177. DOI: 10.1007/s00167-014-2987-4

[89] Vaquerizo V, Padilla S, Aguirre JJ, Begoña L, Orive G, Anitua E. Two cycles of plasma rich in growth factors (PRGF-Endoret) intra-articular injections improve stiffness and activities of daily living but not pain compared to one cycle on patients with symptomatic knee osteoarthritis. Knee Surgery, Sports Traumatology, Arthroscopy. 2018;**26**(9):2615-2621. DOI: 10.1007/s00167-017-4565-z

[90] Sánchez M, Fiz N, Guadilla J, Padilla S, Anitua E, Sánchez P, et al. Intraosseous infiltration of platelet-rich plasma for severe knee osteoarthritis. Arthroscopy Techniques. 2014;**3**(6):e713-e717. DOI: 10.1016/j.eats.2014.09.006

[91] Fiz N, Pérez JC, Guadilla J, Garate A, Sánchez P, Padilla S, et al. Intraosseous infiltration of platelet-rich plasma for severe hip osteoarthritis. Arthroscopy Techniques. 2017;**6**(3):e821-e825. DOI: 10.1016/j.eats.2017.02.014

[92] Sánchez M, Delgado D, Sánchez P, Muiños-López E, Paiva B, Granero-Moltó F, et al. Combination of intra-articular and intraosseous injections of platelet rich plasma for severe knee osteoarthritis: A pilot study. BioMed Research International. 2016;**2016**:4868613. DOI: 10.1155/2016/4868613

[93] Sánchez M, Delgado D, Pompei O, Pérez JC, Sánchez P, Garate A, et al. Treating severe knee osteoarthritis

with combination of intra-osseous and intra-articular infiltrations of platelet-rich plasma: An observational study. Cartilage. 2019;**10**(2):245-253. DOI: 10.1177/1947603518756462

[94] Su K, Bai Y, Wang J, Zhang H, Liu H, Ma S. Comparison of hyaluronic acid and PRP intra-articular injection with combined intra-articular and intraosseous PRP injections to treat patients with knee osteoarthritis. Clinical Rheumatology. 2018;**37**(5):1341-1350. DOI: 10.1007/s10067-018-3985-6

[95] Bastos R, Mathias M, Andrade R, Bastos R, Balduino A, Schott V, et al. Intra-articular injections of expanded mesenchymal stem cells with and without addition of platelet-rich plasma are safe and effective for knee osteoarthritis. Knee Surgery, Sports Traumatology, Arthroscopy. 2018;**26**(11):3342-3350. DOI: 10.1007/s00167-018-4883-9

[96] Bastos R, Mathias M, Andrade R, Amaral RJFC, Schott V, Balduino A, et al. Intra-articular injection of culture-expanded mesenchymal stem cells with or without addition of platelet-rich plasma is effective in decreasing pain and symptoms in knee osteoarthritis: A controlled, double-blind clinical trial. Knee Surgery, Sports Traumatology, Arthroscopy. 2019. DOI: 10.1007/s00167-019-05732-8 [Epub ahead of print]

[97] Gibbs N, Diamond R, Sekyere EO, Thomas WD. Management of knee osteoarthritis by combined stromal vascular fraction cell therapy, platelet-rich plasma, and musculoskeletal exercises: A case series. Journal of Pain Research. 2015;**8**:799-806. DOI: 10.2147/JPR.S92090

[98] Pintat J, Silvestre A, Magalon G, Gadeau AP, Pesquer L, Perozziello A, et al. Intra-articular injection of mesenchymal stem cells and platelet-rich plasma to treat patellofemoral osteoarthritis: Preliminary results of a long-term pilot study. Journal of Vascular and Interventional Radiology. 2017;**28**(12):1708-1713. DOI: 10.1016/j.jvir.2017.08.004

Chapter 4

Regenerative Medicine and Eye Diseases

Enzo Maria Vingolo, Laura Contento, Antonio Florido, Filippo Avogaro and Paolo Giuseppe Limoli

Abstract

The chapter examines the use of stem cells in ophthalmological pathologies affecting both the anterior and posterior segments. The authors review the clinical trials that have most contributed to defining the role and potential of stem cell regenerative therapy in corneal and retinal pathology. The results described in the scientific literature are analyzed and commented, without neglecting the possible side effects related to the use of this therapy. Within the anterior segment, the greatest efforts were made to study the possible uses of limbal epithelial stem cells (LESCs). They were the first stem cells to be discovered at the level of the anterior segment and currently the only ones involved in clinical practice with satisfactory results. At this juncture there have been significant successes in the treatment of corneal stem cell deficiency and of corneal scars. The chapter later investigates the possible applications of stem cell therapy in degenerative retinal diseases, with particular reference to retinitis pigmentosa, Stargardt's disease, and age-related macular degeneration. It then describes how the use of cell therapies, in particular those that use ADSC, can contribute, through various methods, to the containment of the evolution of retinal degenerative diseases. These mechanisms cover various biological aspects and can be summarized as follows: neurotrophism, oxidation, vascular changes, apoptosis, inflammation, or immunology. The ophthalmological modalities of the cell graft and what is the ideal approach for an ophthalmological cellular surgery are later on described. Finally, the technique used by the author and the possible outcomes in the course of degenerative retinopathy are described.

Keywords: ophthalmology, stem cells, regenerative medicine, degenerative diseases

1. Introduction

Regenerative medicine has been a major topic in the last few decades. The use of stem cells has opened up new perspectives in the therapeutic approach to many different diseases. Even in the ophthalmological field, the use of stem cells has allowed an improvement in the clinical outcome of different pathologies such as limbal stem cell deficiency, corneal scarring, retinitis pigmentosa, Stargardt's disease, age-related macular degeneration, and retinal atrophy following various vascular conditions. Many of these pathologies have always been considered untreatable, leading to a progressive sight loss; the arrival of stem cell therapy has led to an entirely new clinical and therapeutic approach to these conditions. Different types of stem cells have been tested as a solution for tissue repair in the different ocular structures.

As for the anterior segment, the most used cells are limbal epithelial stem cells (LESCs), found at the level of the Vogt palisades. As regards the posterior segment, the stem cells used for the treatment of retinal degenerative diseases are embryonic stem cells (ESCs), induced pluripotent stem cells (IPSCs), and mesenchymal stem cells (MSCs).

LESCs: Also known as corneal epithelial stem cells, they are located in the basal epithelial layer of the corneal limbus. They form the border between the cornea and the sclera and are implied in the regular corneal renewal. They are also implied in corneal repair activity after severe damage of corneal surface.

ESCs: The first ESCs were obtained from mouse embryos and immediately showed their ability to express neural markers and to migrate into the retina when applied intravitreally. Also, they seemed to be able to integrate into the retinal layers and act as neuroprotective factors. Clinical trials conducted in the human eyes have demonstrated that the subretinal application of these cells shows no signs of rejection, ectopic tissue development, negative proliferation, or tumor formation in a 1-year follow-up.

IPSCs: These cells are obtained from reprogramming adult somatic fibroblasts through retroviruses or lentiviruses. Compared with ESCs, they show less risk of rejection and less need for immunosuppressive therapy. However, further studies have suggested that IPSCs can stimulate oncogenes/suppress tumor suppressor genes, resulting in gene mutations and malignant transformation. The many molecular passages required for their production also seem to act as a trigger for the genetic instability shown by these cells.

MSCs: These cells are derived from many different tissues (peripheral blood, bone marrow, adipose tissue, cord blood, teeth, central nervous system, and liver). Once acquired, MSCs can be expanded in cell cultures maintaining their stemness. They can differentiate into various cells (mesodermal, ectodermal, and endodermal cells), including neuron-like cells. Since they are capable of secreting neurotrophic factors, repairing neural connections, and stimulating the formation of synapses, MSCs are also appreciated for their "structural" function. Moreover, they have shown a strong immunosuppressive action inhibiting the release of pro-inflammatory cytokines; therefore they allow both autologous and allogenic transplantation. Finally, their use does not seem to be related to tumor formation. For these reasons, researchers look at stem cells as a promising therapeutic option for degenerative retinal diseases. Nevertheless, it must be said that various ocular complications related with the use of these cells have been described (see Section 3).

2. Regenerative medicine in the anterior segment of the eye

Stem cells are unspecialized cells that have been a focal point of the field of regenerative medicine, frequently considered as the future of medicine. The first medical science branch which directly benefits from stem cells for regenerative treatment was ophthalmology. The triumph of regenerative medicine in ophthalmology can be attributed to its accessibility, ease of follow-up, and the eye being an immune-privileged organ. Two key characteristic attributes of stem cells are pluripotency, the capacity to differentiate into multiple lineages, and proliferation. These cells have the ability to replace damaged or diseased cells under certain specific circumstances. Stem cell-based therapy has now reached a state where ocular tissues damaged by disease or injury can be repaired and/or regenerated. The eye is an ideal organ for studying regenerative medicine thanks to the ease of access for the therapeutic procedure as well as its status of being an immune-privileged organ. Such therapy involves various techniques in which stem cells are injected into both the cellular and extracellular matrix microenvironments. Corneal epithelial stem cell transplantation has been the most employed stem cell-based therapy after bone marrow transplantation. Stem cell-based treatment in ophthalmology follows two possible ways: a cell replacement therapy strategy or a strategy involving trophic factor-based guidance cues. Throughout treatment, outcomes are related to different factors like our in-depth knowledge of the disease, the source of stem cells, the plausible mechanism driving the therapeutic outcome, and the mode of treatment. Considering specifically the anterior segment, we will analyze separately stem cell pools of the conjunctiva, the cornea, the trabecular meshwork, and the lens. In addition we will make few words about the iris stem cell pool. This pool also subspecializes in three types of cells with different capacities for multiplication: putative stem cells with high reproductive potential, the generally slow-cycling activity cells, and transit amplifying cells (TAC), which have a reduced reproductive potential but rapid expansion time.

2.1 Conjunctiva

The conjunctiva, apart from being a protection against pathogenic entry, is a connective tissue provided by a high vascularization that offers channels for proper flow of nutrients and fluids. From the anatomical point of view, the conjunctiva is an unkeratinized stratified squamous epithelium, in which goblet cells are also present, that covers the exposed scleral surface (bulbar conjunctiva) and the interior part of the eyelids (tarsal conjunctiva). Conjunctival cells undertake renewal similar to the corneal epithelium, but with a still elusive source of stem cells. Conjunctival stem cells undergo a differentiation pathway that can take them to become either mucin-producing goblet cells or epithelial cells. The dividing basal cell migration starts from the bulbar conjunctiva and takes it to the corneal surface before differentiation. Conjunctival epithelial cells are negative for CK3 and CK12 but positive for CK19. As shown in clonal culture assays, the stem cells located in the fornical niche can differentiate into epithelial cells as well as goblet cells. This provides important evidence that the stem cell pool supporting conjunctival renewal is located in the fornix region. Commitment to differentiate into goblet cells occurs relatively late; in fact goblet cells are generated by stem cell-derived transient amplifying cells. The decision of a conjunctival keratinocyte to differentiate into a goblet cell appears to be dependent upon an intrinsic "cell doubling clock." Ocular processes that affect the cornea also affect the conjunctiva; some examples are conjunctival scarring, cicatricial pemphigoid, thickening, dry eye, or mucin. In order to treat conjunctival stem cell deficiency and scarring, conjunctival autografts, oral mucous membrane grafts, nasal turbinate mucosa grafts, and amniotic membrane are often used. Conjunctival cells cultured on amniotic membrane have been used for cell transplantation in patients with limbal stem cell deficiency (LSCD). Recent patient follow-up reports have shown that transplantation of autologous conjunctival epithelial cells improved the clinical parameters of total LSCD with respect to vision acuity, impression cytology, and in vivo confocal analysis. These cells were cultivated ex vivo on amniotic membrane with the presence of epidermal growth factor, insulin, cholera toxin, and hydrocortisone to produce the corneal lineage; the cells were transplanted after 2 weeks of culture. Ultrathin polymembrane substrate has also been shown to support conjunctival epithelial cell proliferation.

2.2 Cornea

The cornea is at the outermost surface of the eye, and its fundamental characteristic is transparency, which is crucial for vision. It is a clear lens that determines the majority part of the dioptric power of the eye (about 43D). Its normal thickness is between 520 and 540 μm and is composed of five layers which are from the outside to the inside: corneal epithelium, Bowman's layer, corneal stroma, Descemet's membrane, and corneal endothelium. Forty-five million people worldwide are bilaterally blind, and another 135 million have a severe impaired vision defect in both eyes because of loss of corneal transparency. In order to correct this kind of problems, therapies ranging from local medications to corneal transplants, and more recently to stem cell therapy, could be applied. The corneal epithelium is a squamous epithelium that has a constant renewal activity, with a vertical turnover of 7–14 days. The corneal stem cell pool is located in the limbus, at the periphery of the cornea, and these cells are called limbal epithelial stem cells (LESCs). The corneal epithelium has a renewal process which is performed by cells generated at the limbus and, migrating from there, in opposition to other squamous epithelia in which each stem cell has the role of regenerating a limited area of epithelium. In the corneal epithelium, stem cells are located at the corneal periphery in the basal layer of the limbal region, called the palisades of Vogt. These are visualized in small clusters and are strictly associated with the stromal matrix and the basal membrane, thereby assisting in cell-cell, cell extracellular matrix, and paracrine signaling communication. The corneal epithelial basal layer is composed mostly of TAC at various stages of maturity, and this could be demonstrated by their elevated expression of a specific isoform of the transcription factor p63 along with a high nuclear to cytoplasmic ratio. The positivity of ATP-binding cassette subfamily G member 2 (ABCG2) has been detected in LESCs as well as in several other cells located in the suprabasal region of the limbus, and these markers could be used to identify the LESC pool. Some reports also indicate that an RNA binding protein called Musashi-1 can be used to stain LESCs. Corneal stem cells also express some other specific markers, enolase, cytokeratin (CK)19, and vimentin, but do not express CK3, CK12, or connexin 43, which are present only in mature corneal epithelial cells. Stromal multipotent stem cells have been identified and expanded to neurospheres in cultures. Corneal stromal stem cells are located in the anterior region of the stroma adjacent to the basal side of the palisades of Vogt and were identified as a side population using the DNA-binding dye Hoechst 33342. These cells expressed genes encoding ABCG2, Bmi1, CD166, c-kit, Pax6, Six2, and Notch1 similarly as mesenchymal stem cell and corneal early development markers. Corneal stromal stem cells, when differentiated, express keratocyte markers like keratocan, ALDH3A1, CXADR, PTDGS, and PDK4. LESC deficiency, either partial or complete, is pathological and is caused by either chemical or mechanical injury or thermal burns or acquired by diseases like aniridia and Stevens-Johnson syndrome. Treatment of such conditions involves LESCs transplantation therapy. In unilateral cases of ocular disease, LESCs from the healthy eye are expanded ex vivo for therapeutic purposes using specific protocols which involve amniotic membrane or fibrin in the presence or absence of growth-arrested 3T3 fibroblast feeder layers. Taking in consideration non-limbal cell types, cultured oral mucosal cells and conjunctival epithelial cells have been transplanted with success to treat LSCD in humans. The peripheral cornea has been proven to contain a higher density of keratocyte precursors with high proliferative capacity. Restoration of corneal transparency, stromal thickness, and collagen fibril defects have been demonstrated as solvable through the injection of corneal stromal stem cells in mice. If it will be shown as successful, such therapy would eliminate the shortage of corneas from donors needed for transplantations. Although stem cell transplantation is performed worldwide, standardized protocols need to be established because of variability in clinical outcomes. An application example of LESCs transplant could be in patients with LSCD who are suffering from a severe loss of vision and annoying irritation, being also poor candidates for conventional corneal transplant. Hence, new surgical strategies have been devised by transplanting LESCs from an autologous or allogeneic source. When in total LSCD only one eye is involved, the reconstruction of the damaged corneal surface can be effectively performed by the application of conjunctival limbal autograft. Although conjunctival limbal autograft has high success rates, if transplantation is carried out at the acute stage of chemical burns when inflammation remains in "active" stage, the surgical outcome is not satisfactory; this notion has been verified in a rabbit model. The potential risk to the patient's donor eye could be reduced with the application of different techniques: the first alternative is to perform LESCs allograft, in which an allogeneic source of LESCs is derived from either living donors matched with HLA or not matching cadavers. Systemic immunosuppression with cyclosporin A or other agents is necessary because the donor tissue is allogeneic, but this solution is potentially toxic. The success rate of limbal allografts declines with time even with systemic application of cyclosporin A. Elements implicated as factors contributing to the poor prognosis for keratolimbal allografts are keratinization, severe dry eye, chronic inflammation, uncorrected lid, and lid margin abnormalities. A combined immunosuppressive regimen together with a meticulous restoration of the ocular surface defense has been shown to further improve the long-term visual outcome of keratolimbal allografts.

2.3 Trabecular meshwork

The trabecular meshwork is a tissue included between the cornea and the iris in the anterior region that has the role of draining the aqueous fluid. It is divided into three parts which have their characteristic ultrastructures: inner uveal meshwork, corneoscleral meshwork, and juxtacanalicular tissue. Intraocular pressure is determined by the correct balance between aqueous production and outflow; a malfunction in this mechanism is a possible risk factor for the development of glaucoma. Trabecular meshwork cells also are implied in the removal of debris in the circulating aqueous humor. Trabecular meshwork cellular markers are vimentin, non-muscle actin, aquaporin-1, acetylated and acetoacetylated alpha-2 adrenergic receptor, matrix GLA protein, and chitinase-3-like-1. Recently, the isolation, characterization, and specific markers of trabecular meshwork cells have been widely studied. These studies suggest that trabecular meshwork cellular population has properties similar to stem cells, expressing mesenchymal cell-associated markers such as CD73, CD90, and CD105, and they have also the ability to differentiate into adipocytes, osteocytes, and chondrocytes. Moreover, further studies showed that trabecular meshwork cells with mesenchymal phenotype are isolated as a side population or as clones expressing specific stem cell markers, not present in mature cells, such as Notch1, OCT-3/OCT-4, ABCG2, AnkG, and MUC1. These stem cells have the ability to differentiate into the trabecular meshwork lineage expressing CHI3L1, AQP1, and TIMP3 markers that underlies to a phagocytic function. Lowering the intraocular pressure is the aim of treatments for glaucoma. The idea for this came primarily from the observation that trabecular meshwork cell division increased after argon laser trabeculoplasty. Current first-line treatments are topical and oral drugs, argon laser trabeculoplasty, and some surgical approaches. Stem cells isolated from human trabecular meshwork and expanded in vitro showed evidence of the ability to home to mouse trabecular meshwork and differentiate into trabecular meshwork cells in vivo according to recent studies. The expanded trabecular meshwork stem cells expressed the stem cell markers Notch1, ABCG2, and MUC1 and were expressing also the trabecular meshwork marker protein CHI3L1. These trabecular meshwork cells were multipotent and had phagocytic properties. Some groups are working on transplanting trabecular meshwork cells or trabecular meshwork progenitor cells combined with argon laser trabeculoplasty as a novel cell-based therapy for glaucoma.

2.4 Lens

The lens is composed of the lens capsule, epithelium, and fibers and, like the cornea, is transparent. It is hypothesized that lens-specific stem cells reside in the lens capsule, although they have not yet been identified. The most confirmed hypothesis is that this cell pool comes from the ciliary body, which is anatomically close to the lens. It has been demonstrated that lens capsule regeneration occurs in lower vertebrates from cells residing in the ciliary body. According to this fact, the probability that lens stem cells might reside in the lens capsule is high. Lens progenitor cells have been derived from human ESCs as well as from induced pluripotent stem cells (iPSCs). Lens stem cells are presumed to have a significant role in the maintenance of the lens transparency and might be implied in cataractogenesis process or other lens abnormalities.

2.5 Iris

The iris has the anatomical role of dividing the space between the cornea and lens into anterior and posterior halves. The microscopic structure consists of an anterior limiting layer that lines the anterior part of the iris stroma that contains muscles, nerves, and vessels and is posteriorly lined by a layer of pigmented and non-pigmented cells. The stroma and the vascular structure of the iris take embryological origin from the anterior region of the optic cup. Epithelial cells of the iris pigment have the ability to grow in spheres and express markers of neural stem/progenitor cells such as Msi, Nestin, and Pax6. It has been revealed by studies from the mouse iris that these cells can also differentiate both in neuronal and glial lineages and express markers such as Rho, Chx10, Otx2, and Olig2. The iris pigment epithelial cells have the potential to be used in cell-based therapy, but nevertheless not much work on validation and quality assessment has been done. Further studies are needed before iris pigment epithelial cells can be used clinically.

3. Regenerative medicine in the posterior segment of the eye

Considering the posterior segment, the main interest is focused on the retina, the target of regenerative medicine. Retinal anatomy is quite complex, and focusing to the microscopic structure, it can be divided into nine layers of nervous tissue that interfaces with the outermost layer of the pigmented epithelium. From external to internal, there are inner segment/outer segment layer, external limiting membrane, outer nuclear layer, outer plexiform layer, inner nuclear layer, inner plexiform layer, ganglion cell layer, nerve fiber layer, and inner limiting membrane.

Stem cells are immature, undifferentiated, highly proliferative cells which are capable of self-renewing and differentiating into many cell types [1]. Therefore, stem cells represent a potentially endless source of tissue renewal; that is why, in the modern era, stem cell therapy has been considered a valid approach for many different pathologies. Ophthalmologists and researchers were not slow to guess the potential applications of stem cell therapy in various degenerative retinal diseases such as retinitis pigmentosa, age-related macular degeneration, Stargardt's macular dystrophy, and other pathological conditions affecting the posterior pole of the eye, including retinal vascular occlusions [1, 2]. These pathologies are responsible for a progressive decline in visual acuity which, in the case of RP,

Stargardt's disease, and AMD, are due to a constant and irreversible loss of retinal photoreceptors and outer nuclear layers. With such premises, it is easy to imagine a therapeutic approach based on the use of stem cells to restore the lost retinal tissue. Stem cells have shown to be able to perform additional functions, such as nutritional support, apoptosis inhibition, synapse formation, immunoregulation, and neurotrophin secretion [1] and have increased even more the enthusiasm for their application in the ophthalmological field. Furthermore, the use of stem cells in the eye seems to offer numerous advantages: firstly, the amount of stem cells required is relatively low, which implies lower costs than those required for the treatment of other tissues of the human body; secondly, the surgical approach is quite easy and the transplanted cells can be easily monitored with the imaging methods currently used in clinical practice. Finally, the immune privilege of the eye allows avoiding long-term immunosuppressive treatment [1]. Several experimental studies conducted on embryonic stem cells (ESCs), induced pluripotent stem cells (IPSCs), or mesenchymal stem cells (MSCs) have demonstrated that they tend to adapt to the retinal environment and can differentiate not only into photoreceptors and RPE cells but also into Müller, amacrine, bipolar, horizontal, and glial cells [1]. Retinitis pigmentosa represented one of the first targets of stem cell therapy in the ophthalmological area: pioneering animal studies have shown that pluripotent stem cells, when placed in murine retinitis pigmentosa models, are able to survive, multiplicate, differentiate, organize into, and function as photoreceptor cells, developing a retina-like organizational structure [3]; using mouse models, Singh et al. have established that at a stage when all host rod cells are lost, transplanted rod precursors can lead to the re-establishment of a proper, correctly polarized outer nuclear layer, indicating that stem cells may recreate a light-sensitive cell layer de novo and restore structurally damaged visual circuits. It has to be said that current methods for photoreceptor derivation from human pluripotent stem cells require long periods of culture and are often inefficient. Boucherie et al. [4] reported that formation of a transient self-organized neuroepithelium from human embryonic stem cells cultured together with extracellular matrix can induce a rapid conversion into retinal progenitors, which are capable of subsequently differentiating into photoreceptor precursors in only 10 days and later acquire rod cell identity within 4 weeks.

Following such promising results, the first phase I/II clinical trials in humans were approved in the United States in 2010; hESC-derived retinal pigment epithelium cells were transplanted into the eyes of patients with Stargardt's macular dystrophy and dry age-related macular degeneration [5]. During differentiation, the stem cells "displayed typical RPE behavior and integrated into the host RPE layer forming mature quiescent monolayers" [5]; after surgery, structural exams showed that cells had attached and persisted during the study. An improvement in best corrected visual acuity was reported both in the patient affected by Stargardt's macular dystrophy and in the patient affected by dry AMD. And what is more important, in 4 months of follow-up, clinicians did not identify signs of hyperproliferation, abnormal growth, ectopic tissue development, or immune-mediated rejection [1, 5], which represent the main concern about stem cell therapy. These findings support the safety of ESC-derived stem cells [1, 6].

Since they are autologous, IPSCs (obtained from reprogramming adult somatic fibroblast cells using retroviruses or lentiviruses) seem to have an even lower risk of rejection. However, because of their abnormal genetic composition, the risk of T cell-mediated immune response or oncogenesis should not be underestimated. In 2015, in fact, a Japanese study on IPSCs that was being conducted on human retinas was interrupted because of a new genetic mutation that occurred in the IPSCs of one of the patients.

MSCs can differentiate into mesodermal, ectodermal, and endodermal cells and can be obtained from many different tissues, including cord and peripheral blood, teeth, central nervous system, liver, bone marrow, and adipose tissue [1]. Several studies have demonstrated that MSCs can easily turn into neuron-like cells and repair damaged cells through a paracrine action which results in a neuroprotective function. In rats, subretinal transplant of MSCs led to their differentiation into different retinal cell types. These results encouraged clinical trials on humans. In a study, Park et al. [2] isolated CD34+ cells from bone marrow and injected it intravitreally. They enrolled six patients affected by dry AMD, retinitis pigmentosa, or retinal vascular diseases. Follow-up included serial ophthalmic examinations, perimetry and/or microperimetry, fluorescein angiography, ERG, and OCT. After 6 months of follow-up, there was no evidence of worsening neither in BCVA nor in full-field ERG. No signs of intraocular inflammation were observed. Other studies on MSCs confirmed their safety in terms of hyperproliferation and systemic side effects. However, as reported, further MSC applications led to other sight-threatening intraocular complications such as elevated intraocular pressure, vitreous hemorrhages, tractional and rhegmatogenous retinal detachment, development of preretinal and vitreal fibrous tissue, and shallowing of the anterior chamber.

Retinal pigment epithelium replacement represents a promising evolution of stem cell therapy. The outer segments of photoreceptors have a very high metabolic demand and undergo a daily renewal; in the healthy retina, the apical processes of the RPE envelope the outer segments of rods and cones, which contain visual pigment, resulting in a diurnal outer segment recycling. Pathological conditions such as drusen deposits, accumulation of lipofuscin, or ischemic insult can result in a disruption of RPE, slowing photoreceptor metabolism and leading to cellular damage. RPE was one of the first tissues to be differentiated in vitro. Nowadays, there are many ongoing clinical trials for pluripotent stem cell-derived RPE replacement. The success of RPE replacement can be explained by various factors: for a start, RPE cell biology and phenotypes are precisely described and conserved among species [7]; the differentiation of embryonic stem cells into RPE cells follows default pathways that are well characterized; animal models of RPE dysfunction are easily available; the amount of RPE required to functionally restore affected retinas is relatively small compared with photoreceptors [7]; and the RPE layers within the retina can be easily visualized using optical coherence tomography, adaptive optics scanning laser ophthalmoscopy, and fundus image. Moreover, studies on animal models have established that sheet transplantation is much more beneficial and effective than single-cell suspension [7], making retinal patches a fascinating approach to degenerative retinal diseases. However, further studies have proven this technique unsuccessful in human models. Nevertheless, studies on retinal sheet transplantation are still ongoing.

Retinal tissue engineering is another intriguing idea for treating late-stage retinal conditions, but various technical and biological issues coming from lab-grown neuroretinal tissue design still need to be solved before it can work in clinics. The size of 3D retinal tissue derived from human pluripotent stem cells is much smaller than that required to obtain a significant clinical outcome, and the implantation of a single piece of retinal organoid may not result in an appreciable improvement in visual acuity in humans [8]. Because of their plasticity, human pluripotent stem cells make an extraordinary source for regenerative medicine. The current challenges of retinal tissue engineering include establishing reproducible protocols for the creation of retinal organoids from stem cells, producing larger pieces of retinal tissue from stem cells along with quality supporting biomaterials, improving surgical methods of delivering retinal organoids into subretinal space, and finding biomaterials to facilitate the survival and functional integration of hPSC-derived grafts into the host's synaptic environment [8].

In conclusion, pioneering studies conducted on animal models have provided hopeful evidence for the hypothesis that stem cell therapy is a valid approach to sight-threatening degenerative retinal diseases, including retinitis pigmentosa, Stargardt's disease, dry age-related macular degeneration, and vascular occlusions. A number of phase I/II clinical trials on humans seem to have confirmed the effectiveness of this method. We now know for sure that when placed in an appropriate tissue niche stem cells not only survive and proliferate but are capable of differentiating into proper retinal cells which exhibit functional characteristics of real photoreceptors, resulting in the development of a retina-like structure [9]. Further studies are needed to put such promising experimental data into clinical practice and establish standardized procedures for the application of stem cell therapy in the ophthalmological field.

4. Cell therapy and atrophic retinal diseases: our experience

Visually impaired patients are affected by a series of different neuroretinal diseases that can target nerve cells such as ganglion cells (RCG), photoreceptors, or support cells such as retinal pigment epithelium cells (RPE). The evolution of these pathologies leads to serious impairment of vision. There are many types of retinal degenerative diseases, including glaucoma, hereditary retinal dystrophy such as retinitis pigmentosa (RP) or Stargardt's disease, age-related macular degeneration (AMD), degenerative myopia, and diabetic retinopathy (DR). In each of these pathologies, regardless of its nature, a certain sequence of molecular events gradually leads to the death of retinal cells.

These mechanisms cover various biological aspects and can be summarized as follows:

- Neurotrophic aspects
- Oxidative aspects
- Vascular alterations
- Apoptosis
- Inflammation and para-inflammation [10, 11]

The sequence can begin with oxidation, photooxidation, or photosensitivity. This is followed by the release of oxidizing substances and free radicals in the cellular environment which in turn causes lipid peroxidation, oxidation of the critical bonds in the protein chains and rupture in those of the DNA, activation of the endogenous nuclease, inhibition of the expression of the Bcl2 gene, and priming of mechanisms of cell apoptosis.

In physiological conditions, healthy retinal cells possess an arsenal of substances with protective action, including antioxidant systems (e.g., SOD) and enzymes, which serve to balance oxidants and free radicals, minimizing damage. One of the best known mechanisms to block or procrastinate apoptotic processes is the activation of the Bc12 gene by growth factors, thus avoiding the fate of death, regardless of the triggering cause. There are cells such as Müller cells or RPE cells, capable of producing, under hypoxic conditions, angiogenic and neurotrophic factors such as FGF and VEGF in order to counterbalance the insult, provided that it is transient [12]. In the case of cellular imbalance, for example, for genetic or inflammatory reasons, for reduction of the chorioretinal blood flow or when a large part of the cells has undergone apoptosis and death with consequent induction of a chronic para-inflammatory condition, the trigger of neuroretinal pathologies, or their progression, can occur. In our opinion, it is possible to apply a therapy aimed at reducing the impact and progression of the disease based on these mechanisms. The therapeutic aim is to slow down or prevent the death of residual retinal cells [13, 14], highlighting the possible efficacy of cell therapy on neurotrophic pathologies of the retina. Currently, in the presence of a dystrophic pathology responsible for a low vision condition, the patient can resort to visual rehabilitation using magnifying aids or filters to improve contrast. In a smaller number of centers, it is possible to benefit from therapies based on the neuromodulation of visual signals, in order to improve not only the image on the retina but also the perception of the same at the cortical level.

However, the progressive loss of photoreceptors contributes to reducing the performance obtained with visual rehabilitation, and the social impact of the progressive loss of functional autonomy should not be underestimated. New therapeutic approaches to neuroretinal degenerations for therapy include restoring defective genes, when the disease is caused by a genetic defect, and transplanting stem cells to replace or repair defective or dead cells, regardless of the cause [15, 16]. Gene therapy is a causal therapy but is currently not clinically available, and the therapeutic results obtained experimentally are still marginal in vivo. For this reason, the interest of the scientific community is also addressed to stem cell-based repair strategies, consisting in the systemic or local injection of stem/progenitor cells for the treatment of multiple chronic pathologies [15, 16]. Stem cells are undifferentiated cells that have the ability to self-renew and differentiate into mature cells. On this basis, cell replacement therapy has been evaluated in recent years as a viable alternative for various pathologies. This therapy hypothesizes the generation of retinal cells from stem cells to replace damaged cells in the diseased retina. This goal can be achieved by releasing embryonic stem cells (ESCs), induced pluripotent stem cells (iPSCs), and mesenchymal stem cells (MSCs) [17] in specific target positions of the eye. Stem cell therapy opens up the possibility of replacing or regenerating the cells now destroyed during the most common neurodystrophic diseases of the retina. However, ESC and iPCS have generated much controversy over ethical, immunological, and oncological issues. Instead, the use of MSC appears to be free from these concerns. The reparative therapy operated by the implanted cells aims to create better conditions for the viability of the residual cells, preventing or slowing their decline. We could therefore define cell therapy, or mediated cell therapy, or any therapeutic modality based on the use of cell grafts that aim not only at the neuroenhancement of compromised cells and the possible regeneration of some elements (such as receptors, mitochondrial components, connection fibers) but also to their integration with the above cells. It remains to be asked whether it is easier to preserve or promote the survival and function of diseased cells than to actively restore retinal cells after they have disappeared following the disease.

4.1 Mesenchymal stem cells as a therapeutic tool

MSCs are characterized by a panel of superficial cell markers proposed by the International Society for Cellular Therapy in 2006. The MSC population is defined as positive over 95% for CD105, CD73, and CD90 and negative over 95% for CD45, CD34, CD14 or CD11b, CD79α or CD19, and HLA-DR [18]. Some molecules present on the surface of MSCs and endothelial cells, such as P-selectin and integrins, let the MSCs themselves migrate to the lesion sites, following their intravascular administration. After joining the endothelium, the MSCs are able to cross it in a metal-dependent way. MSCs are obtainable from umbilical cord blood, peripheral blood, bone marrow, and adipose tissue. MSCs are multipotent: appropriate culture conditions associated with specific growth factors drive the differentiation of MSCs into specific cell types and can differentiate into various cell types, including osteocytes, adipocytes, vascular endothelial cells, cardiomyocytes, pancreatic beta cells, and hepatocytes. Therefore, MSCs play a key role in organogenesis, remodeling, and tissue repair. Experimental studies have also reported that MSCs have the potential to differentiate into retinal progenitor cells, photoreceptors, and retinal neuron-like cells. Furthermore, stem cells, in particular mesenchymal stem cells (MSCs), are able to perform multiple functions, such as immunoregulation, anti-apoptosis of neurons, and neurotrophin secretion, and the current opinion is that MSCs can exert neuroprotective and proregenerative effects, through the secretion of factors that act in a paracrine way. An increasing number of studies also report that MSCs are capable of giving rise to neuron-like cells. Not only are they able to differentiate into neurons for cell replacement therapy but to maintain and regulate the microenvironment through paracrine effects by modulating the plasticity of damaged host tissues [19, 20].

Of all the MSC collection sites, adipose tissue is particularly interesting and rich in stem cells derived from fat, called ADSCs [21]. These cells are able to secrete neurotrophic growth factors and promote survival, restore the release of the synaptic transmitter, integrate into existing neural and synaptic networks, and re-establish functional connections [22]. ADSCs produce bFGF, vascular endothelial growth factor (VEGF), macrophage colony stimulating factor (M-CSF), granulocyte-macrophage colony stimulating factor (GM-CSF), placental growth factor (PlGF), the transforming growth factor (TGFβ), hepatocyte growth factor (HG), insulin growth factor (IGF-1), interleukin (IL) and angiogenin, ciliary neurotrophic factor (CNTF), and the brain-derived neurotrophic factor (BDNF). Another type of mesenchymal tissue is represented by adipose tissue which, just like the bone marrow, contains a large population of stem cells within its stromal compartment. Stromal adipocytes or fat stromal cells secrete a series of hormones, factors, and protein signals, called adipokines, which are associated with the role of the adipocyte in energy homeostasis. Fat cells produce the base fibroblast growth factor (bFGF), the epidermal growth factor (EGF), the insulin-like growth factor-1 (IGF-1), the interleukin (IL), the transforming growth-β (TGFβ), the pigmented epithelium-derived factor (PEDF), and adiponectin. Another type of cell of mesenchymal origin is the platelet, originating from the subdivision of megakaryocytes. Platelets, normally known for their hemostatic action, also release substances that promote tissue repair, angiogenesis, and inflammation modulation. In addition, they induce cell migration and adhesion at angiogenesis sites, as well as the differentiation of endothelial progenitors into mature endothelial cells. Platelets produce platelet-derived growth factor (PDGF), IGF-1, TGFβ, VEGF, bFGF, EGF, platelet-derived angiogenesis factor (PDAF), and thrombospondin (TSP) [23].

The therapeutic potential of mesenchymal cells is based on the stabilizing effect against the retinal cells exerted by the cytokines and the growth factors released paracrinically when they are grafted. The binding of the growth factor to the specific surface receptor placed on the cytoplasmic membrane of the target cell is the initial step that triggers a cascade of events, activating particular second messengers that guarantee the signal transduction at the intracellular level. The ultimate goal is the regulation of enzyme activity or gene expression (**Figure 1**) [24, 25]. In particular, activated transcription factors, entering the nucleus and binding directly or indirectly to DNA, regulate the expression of various genes with

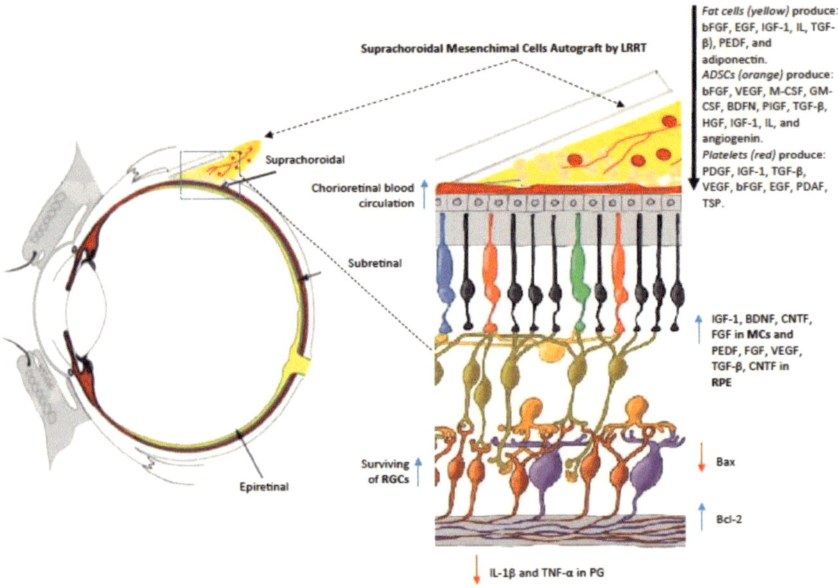

Figure 1.
The growth factors produced by mesenchymal cells implanted in the suprachoroidal space can act both directly on the retinal cells and indirectly, through the mediation of Müller (MC) and RPE cells, generating angiotrophic, neurotrophic, anti-inflammatory, and antiapoptotic effects [26, 27]. Image courtesy of P. Limoli-Milan Low Vision Study Center.

different mechanisms, promoting greater synthesis of proteins including enzymes and cytokines. These end products play a key role in cell survival, as assessed by the improvement in electrical activity recorded by ERG [27]. The growth factors are essential to trigger the cell transition from G0 or resting phase to G1 or growth phase. Furthermore these molecules stimulate a wide range of cellular processes, including mitosis, cell survival, migration, and cellular differentiation.

4.2 Pathophysiological co-factoriality and cell therapy

The grafting of mesenchymal cells into the suprachoroidal space promotes a continuous paracrine increase in GF that can positively interfere with the evolution of retinal diseases in several ways.

Therapeutic activity can be classified into:

1. Hemorheological activity

2. Antioxidative activity

3. Anti-inflammatory activity

4. Antiapoptotic activity

5. Cytoprotective activity

6. Therapeutic synergy with electrical stimulation (ES)

It is worth noting that the boundaries between these categories are not necessarily defined. The hemorheological activity and its increase help to restore an effective retinal perfusion. Photoreceptor loss that occurs in retinal diseases has been identified as the cause of microvascular dysfunction due to the release of cellular waste secondary to apoptosis. In fact, there is a correlation between the extent of the blood flow and the evolutionary stage of the atrophic pathology, in a vicious circle that leads to the final loss of other photoreceptors. Several factors such as VEGF, bFGF, angiogenin, PDAF, PIGF, PDGF, EGF, and TGF-β have been shown to promote endothelial regeneration and therefore can contribute to the reperfusion of the choriocapillaris. Furthermore, others, including TSP and PEDF, inhibit pathological neovascular processes [28, 29]. Antioxidative activity prevents oxygen-induced photoreceptor cell death. One of the underlying causes of photoreceptor deterioration, which may explain the evolution of retinal degeneration, is hyperoxia which results in a more intense oxidation process and in the formation of reactive oxygen species (ROS). Excessive generation of reactive oxygen species causes damage to membrane lipoproteins and cellular DNA, thus leading to apoptosis and the death of photoreceptors [30]. The mechanism involved in hyperoxia can be illuminated by the excessive amount of oxygen in the choroid, similar to the arterial oxygen level, which results from the deterioration and death of the photoreceptor, in addition to foveal exposure to light and the concomitant lack of anti-enzyme oxidants, such as superoxide dismutase (SOD), glutathione-peroxidase, and catalases, normally expressed in the mitochondria of the internal segments of the cone and capable of catalyzing the decomposition of hydrogen peroxide into water and oxygen molecules [31]. The concentration of bFGF within photoreceptors has been shown to increase in response to stress in order to promote retinal cell survival and prevent oxygen-induced photoreceptor cell death [32, 33]. Anti-inflammatory activity can counteract the negative effects induced by microglial activation, which occurs as soon as the apoptotic processes induced by retinal degeneration begin [34, 35]. In turn, the apoptosis and death of photoreceptors are suggested by the ignition of an inflammatory microclimate that supports the chronicity and progression of a large number of neurodegenerative diseases. In particular, RPE performs a series of essential processes for homeostasis and retinal function and constitutes the front of the immune defense of the retina: RPE cells are able to secrete a diversified panel of pro-inflammatory cytokines, for example, IL-6, IL-8, chemoattractant monocyte protein-1 (MCP-1), and interferon-β (IFN-β), as well as anti-inflammatory factors, e.g., IL-11 and TGF-β. Intravitreal administration of MSC has been shown to exert a significant effect on the host's immune response by suppressing the production of pro-inflammatory cytokines, such as IFN-β and TNF-α through IL-1 receptor antagonist (IL-1RA) and prostaglandin E2 receptor (PGE2R) activation [36]. The therapeutic effect of MSCs is corroborated by the neurotrophic action of ciliary neurotrophic factor (CNTF) and brain-derived neurotrophic factor (BDNF): in culturing retinal ganglion cells, under conditions of oxidative stress, MSC expels the last factor that helps reduce pro-inflammation cytokine release, e.g., tumor necrosis factor-α (TNF-α) and interleukin-1 (IL-1) [33]. M-CSF, GM-CSF, and IL exercise an anti-inflammatory function and recruit macrophages by chemotaxis that help remove intraretinal cell debris [37]. The antiapoptotic activity is regulated by cytokines with an inhibiting (antiapoptotic) or inducing apoptosis (pro-apoptotic) action [38].

Proteins of the Bcl-2 family are particularly known for their regulation of apoptosis by interacting with caspases, a family of cysteine-containing protease enzymes (proteinases or caspases specific to cysteine's aspartate). RPE and Müller cells produce a wide heterogeneity of factors, e.g., fibroblast growth factors (FGF-1, FGF-2, and FGF-5), transforming growth factor-β (TGF-β), insulin-like growth factor 1 (IGF-1), ciliary neurotrophic factor (CNTF), platelet-derived growth factor (PDGF), vascular endothelial growth factor (VEGF), some members of the Interleukin family, and the pigmented epithelium factor (PEDF). This multitude of growth factors, released in the retinal cytosol, is able to produce a wide trophic action on adjacent structures. As a consequence, the progressive loss of RPE and Müller cells hinders the incretion of these bioactive agents: their antiapoptotic action is therefore slowed down or completely blocked. The administration of mesenchymal cells can interfere with the apoptotic process involved in retinal degeneration. The growth factors excreted by the grafted mesenchymal cells perform a variety of functions; in particular they are able to facilitate the expression of the Bcl-2 gene in order to avoid the inexorable death of the cells, regardless of the root causes [17]. The cytoprotective activity of the GF contributes to neuroprotection by regulating the metabolic activity of the photoreceptors, which is widely compromised in diseases of the retina. Like bFGF, PEDF has been found to exert neurotrophic activity, inducing the overall survival of photoreceptors [39]. Significant data currently exist to suggest that certain factors such as EGF play a role in potentiating the neuroprotective action of Müller cells by stimulating their intracellular transcription and bFGF expression [40]. The VEGF released by the PRP has been shown to stimulate the proliferation of ADSCs which therefore promote the survival of grafted autologous fat and adipocytes [41]. BFGF is known to directly promote the survival of photoreceptors [42]. Synergy with electrical stimulation (ES) addresses four main aspects: survival of native cells, survival of transplanted cells, integration of transplanted cells, and functional formation of synapses/axon regeneration [43]. In recent years, the synergy between cell therapies and electrical stimulation has started to be considered as a possible treatment for degenerative diseases. Rat retinas treated with ES showed a reduction in apoptosis [44]. It has also been shown that in light-induced retinal degeneration models, stimulation with ES contains the death of photoreceptors and preserves the length of the external segment [45]. Consequently, it can be assumed that ES treatment can create a more balanced and less hostile environment by modifying the secretion of neurotrophic factors. ES affects the upregulation of neurotrophic factors in Müller cells normally involved in this protection mechanism. After ES, increased expression of in vivo beta fibroblast growth factor (b-FGF), insulin growth factor 1 (IGF-1), and brain-derived neurotrophic factor (BDNF) was observed. Conversely, ES reduces the production of pro-inflammatory cytokines such as tumor necrosis factor-α (TNF-α), interleukin-1β (IL-1β), and the pro-apoptotic gene Bax. The release of neurotrophic factors from the postsynaptic membrane made possible by neuromodulation, together with the enrichment of the same factors in the extracellular environment managed by autologous grafts, determines the formation of synapses at a presynaptic level, facilitating and strengthening neurotransmission [44, 45].

4.3 Cell therapy and routes of administration

The effectiveness of cellular treatments for atrophic pathologies of the retina, in order to stabilize and enhance the visual function, is based on two key elements: on the one hand, the surgical implant techniques and the cell lines used, and on the other by the quantity and quality of residual retinal cells, in other words from the earliness of the treatment. The technique must be simple, totally risk-free, and painless, and the exploited cells must not cause further damage to the residual retinal cell or to the person. Cytokines and growth factors, released paracrinically from the cells administered, must bind to membrane receptors to trigger the pathway of intracellular signal transduction. They still require retinal cells that are still alive.

From the studies carried out so far, it seems that the greater the number of residual cells, the greater the interaction between GF and chorioretinal cell membrane receptors, cellular activity, and, ultimately, the improvement of visual performance (VP) [27]. The release of growth factors in a retina with very low

DOI: http://dx.doi.org/10.5772/intechopen.92749

cellularity hardly causes detectable neuroenhancement. To achieve this goal, different approaches have been explored by inserting these cells in the subtenonian space and in the intravitreal or subretinal space. But it seems that positioning the implant in the suprachoroidal space can satisfy efficacy and safety. In fact, the graft under the tenon, although it has therapeutic significance, does not allow the growth factors produced to reach the neuroretinal tissues inside the sclera in important quantities.

Intravitreal injections of cellular material are effective and simple to perform, but it is necessary to pierce the bulb and leave this material free in the vitreous chamber. Serious complications such as infection, vitreoretinal tractions, and bleeding are also possible.

The release in the subretinal area seems to be the best for the possibility of a potential modification of cell lines due to the direct contact of MSCs with neuronal cells, but their grafting is even more dangerous when the retina is compromised by atrophic diseases [46]. The suprachoroidal graft maximizes the supply of growth factors that flow directly to the choroidal level and through the choroid to the entire retina without creating bulbar perforation. In our experience, in order to have the therapeutic action of growth factors in the retinal environment, we have explored the possibility of treating the dystrophic retina with the implantation of the cell types of mesenchymal origin mentioned above, in detail adipose stromal cells (ASC), stem cells derived from adipose tissue (ADSC) contained in the stromal-vascular fraction (SVF) of adipose tissue, and platelets (PLT) recovered in platelet-rich plasma (PRP) [47–49]. To this end, we used a surgical technique called Limoli retinal restoration technique (LRRT), described in previous works (**Figure 2**) [27, 50, 51]. The autotransplantation of ADSC, ACS, and PLT above the choroid plane improves the incretion of the bioactive factors produced in the choroidal flow and, consequently, promotes their widespread diffusion through the

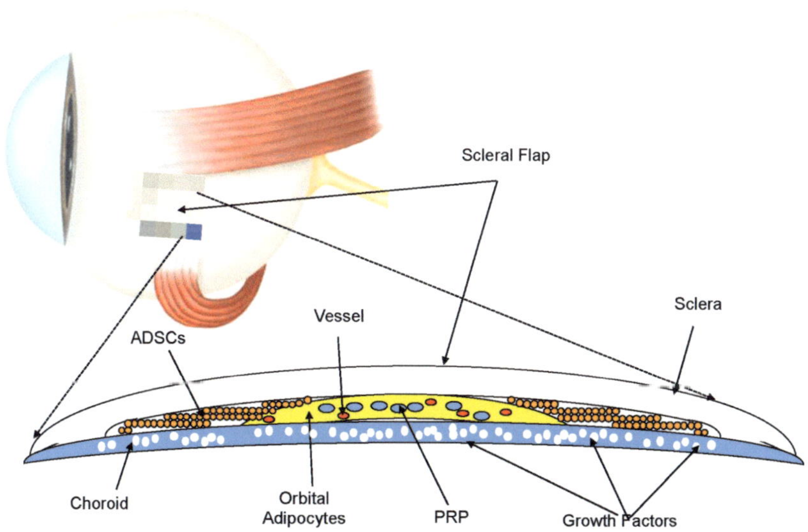

Figure 2.
Autotransplantation of adipose tissue, ADSCs from vascular-stromal fraction, and PRP according to the Limoli retinal restoration technique (LRRT). The production of growth factors (GF), characteristic of these cells, is poured directly into the choroidal flow in paracrine mode, helping to maintain the trophism of the retinal cells. The GF, through the choroidal flux, have a direct action on the choroid, on the Müller cells, on the RPE cells with improvement of the physiology of the external segments (OS), on the rods, and on the cones. Image courtesy of P. Limoli-Milan Low Vision Center.

retinal tissue, finally exuding in the vitreous body. This action positively influences some functional parameters after interaction with the residual cells.

The relapses of cell therapy favor a better choroidal perfusion and a higher trophism of the photoreceptors, both directly (GF) and mediated by the RPE and Müller cells. It is therefore believed that the interaction between retinal cells and growth factors plays a crucial role in leading to an improvement in the prospects of degenerative retinopathy, to prevent and/or delay its progression.

The possible goals with cell therapy are schematically:

- Restoration and neuroenhancement on residual cells (**Figure 3**)
- The partial reduction of the scotoma (**Figure 4**)
- The improvement of the reading performance by stabilizing the fixation obtained with neuroenhancement (**Figure 5**)
- The improvement of the choroidal flow (**Figure 6**)
- The conservation of useful areas such as the fovea (when it is still present) or the preferential reading field (**Figure 7**)
- The slowing down of retinal disease (**Figure 8**)

In our study, greater foveal or retinal thickness is associated with a better prognosis. On the other hand, the lack of cells cannot make interactions between growth factors and membrane receptors possible [27, 51]. For this reason, cell therapies

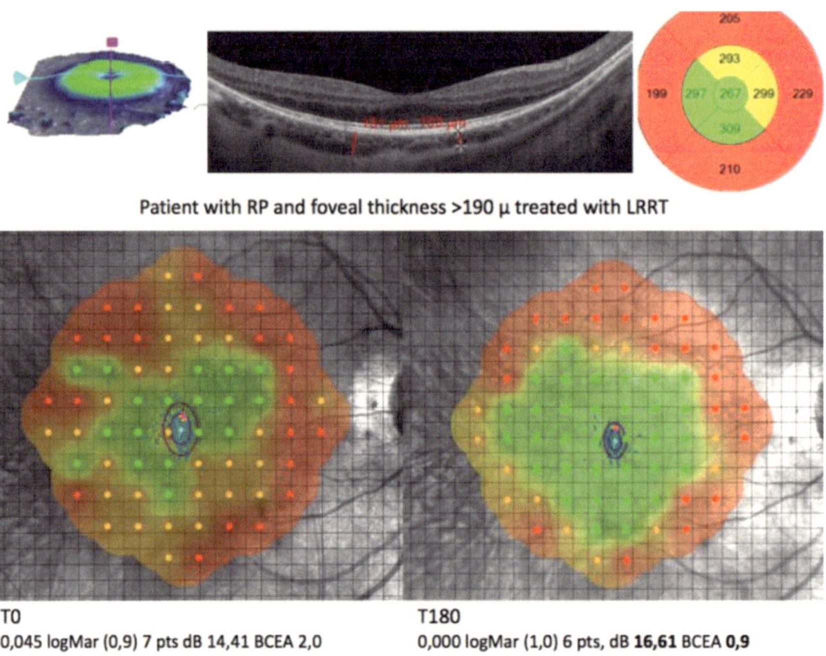

Figure 3.
The image shows the effect of a suprachoroidal implantation of autologous mesenchymal cells in a patient with retinitis pigmentosa. The wealth of cells in the foveal area, documented by OCT, and therefore the high number of interactions between growth factors produced and specific membrane receptors, has allowed (T180) an increase in visual performance (BCVA, dB, pts). Image courtesy of P. Limoli-Milan Studies Center.

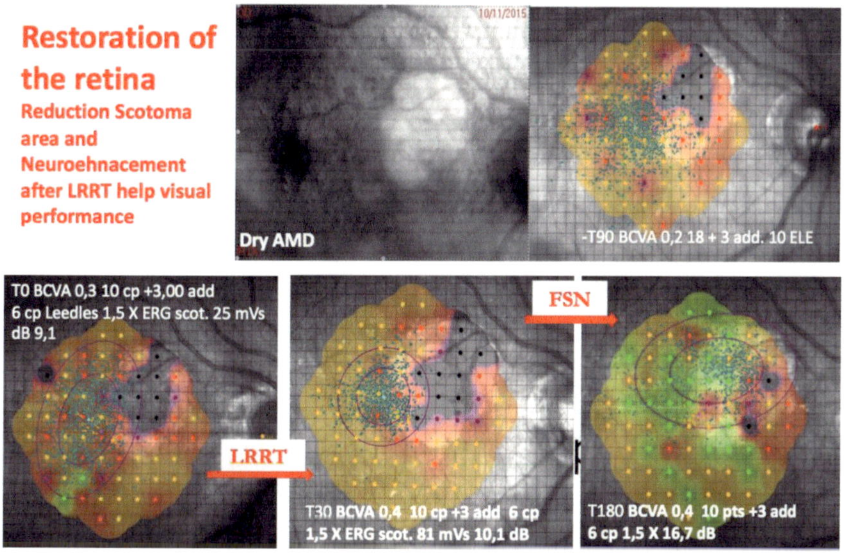

Figure 4.
Patient suffering from dry AMD with areolar evolution (retinography top left). The patient treated for 3 months with supplements did not show any increase in sensitivity even if we recorded a near viscous increase (picture below left). After suprachoroid implantation of autologous mesenchymal cells (T30 and T180), we observed an increase in sensitivity outside the atrophic area and a further improvement in the visual acuity. The near vision passes from 18 points of the initial evaluation to 10 points of the final evaluation which took place 9 months later. Image courtesy of P. Limoli-Milan Low Vision Center.

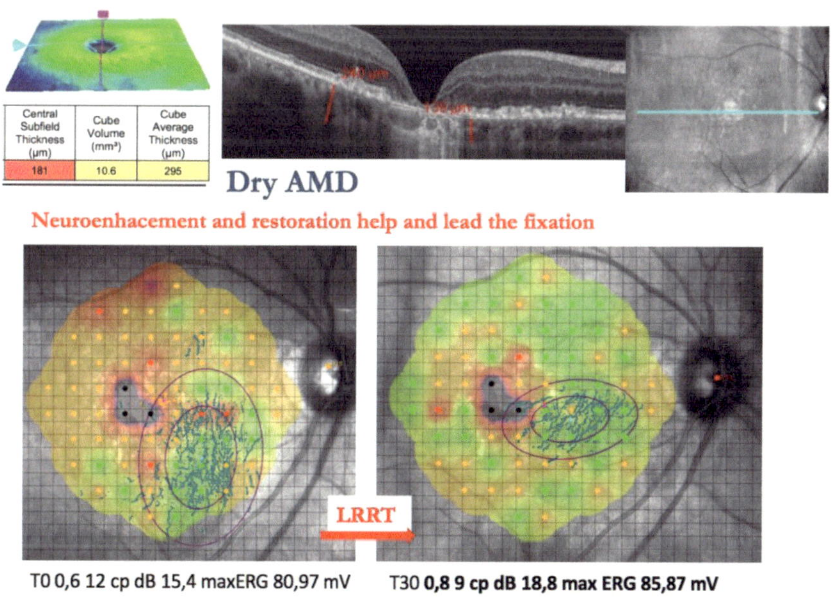

Figure 5.
The figure shows a case of dry AMD with a small atrophic area. An autologous suprachoroidal implant was performed and from the first month (bottom right) an improvement in visual performance was observed in terms of sensitivity, electrical activity, and visual acuity for far and near. Retinal neuroenhancement favored the re-centering and stabilization of fixations. Image courtesy of P. Limoli-Milan Low Vision Center.

must be proposed as soon as the disease starts to progress, when the cells are still numerous and the patient realizes the functional change. If a disease is stable and its impact on vision is accepted by the patient, it is not advisable to propose cellular

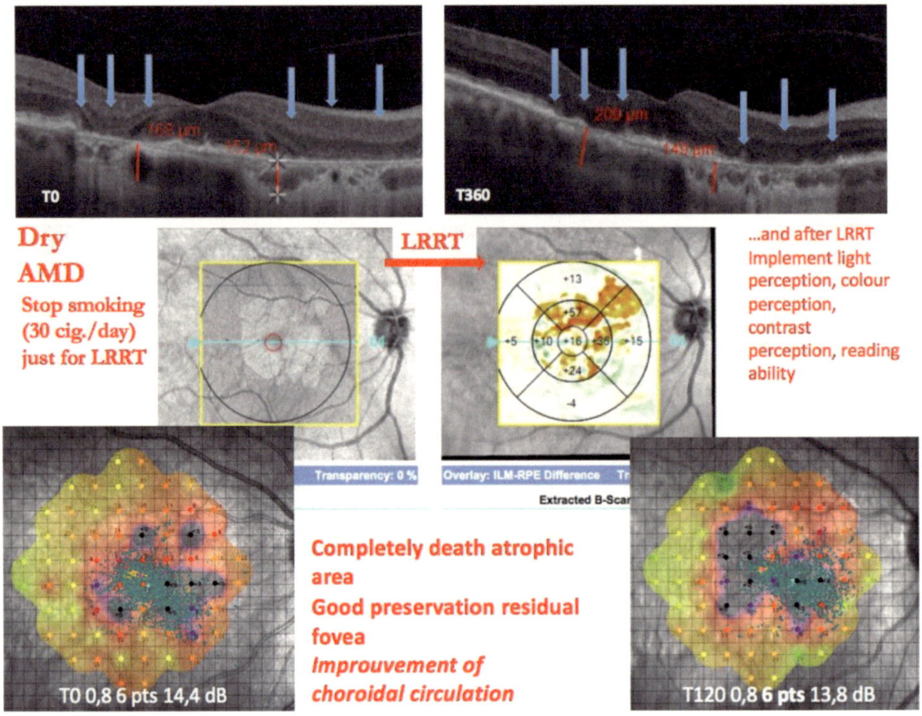

Figure 6.
Patient suffering from dry AMD with a peripheral areolar evolution (blue arrows at the top left). Sensitivity appears to be compromised by a paracentral scotoma, but survival of the fovea allows for good visual ability (bottom left). After autologous suprachoroidal graft of mesenchymal cells (T180), we observed an increase in the thickness of the choroid (top right and center right). Despite the increase in the paracentral scotoma which has become more profound as an expression of a now dying area, the improvement of the choroidal circulation has contributed to the maintenance of the foveal area and the stabilization of visual performance. Image courtesy of P. Limoli-Milan Low Vision Center.

surgery. Knowledge of the overall amount of retinal cells is of particular importance: the rehabilitator and surgeon should be aware of this as a precise predictor of outcome for patients treated with cell therapy.

5. Conclusions

Stem cell therapy is going to change the natural history of various ophthalmologic conditions. For example, several studies have highlighted the chance to repair corneal damage through the implantation of conjunctival cells grown on the amniotic membrane with a good clinical outcome. In addition, an improvement in clinical parameters was observed in patients with limbal stem cell deficiency through the implantation of autologous conjunctival stem cells. This is evidenced by an increase in the visual acuity and a reduction of irritation. Despite biochemical evidences of the existence of stem cell populations in the remaining portions of the anterior segment (trabecular, iris, and crystalline), their clinical use is still under study.

Pioneering studies conducted on animal models have provided hopeful evidence for the hypothesis that stem cell therapy is a valid approach to sight-threatening degenerative retinal diseases, including retinitis pigmentosa, Stargardt's disease, dry age-related macular degeneration, and vascular occlusions. A number of phase I/II clinical trials on humans seem to have confirmed the effectiveness

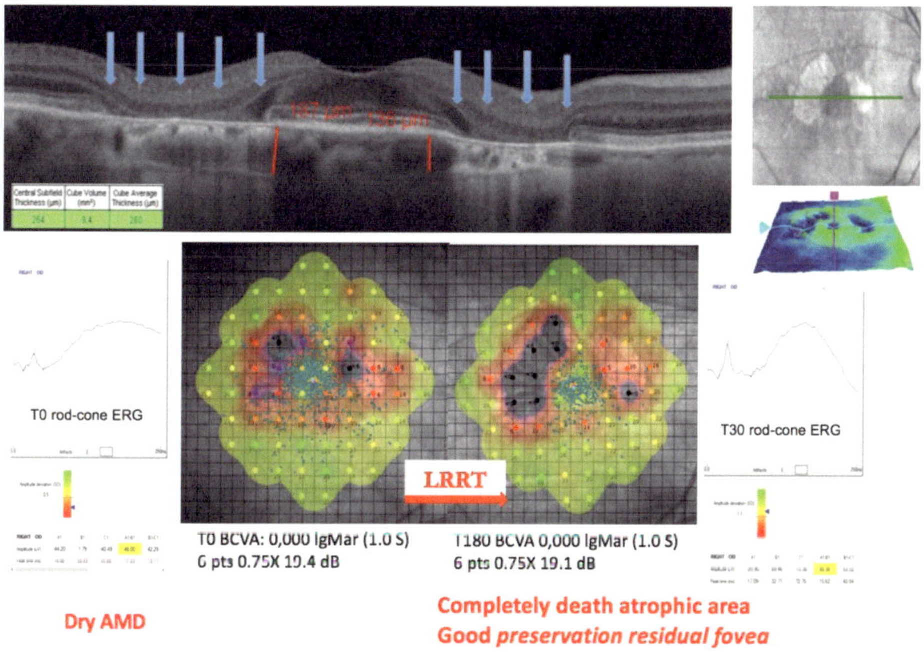

Figure 7.
Another case of dry AMD with saving of the foveal area (above) and T0. Six months after LRRT, despite the progression of the scotoma within the paracentral atrophic areas, the fovea has maintained its sensitivity, and visual performance has been preserved (T180). ERG activity (bottom left) showed an increase (bottom right). Image courtesy of P. Limoli-Milan Low Vision Center.

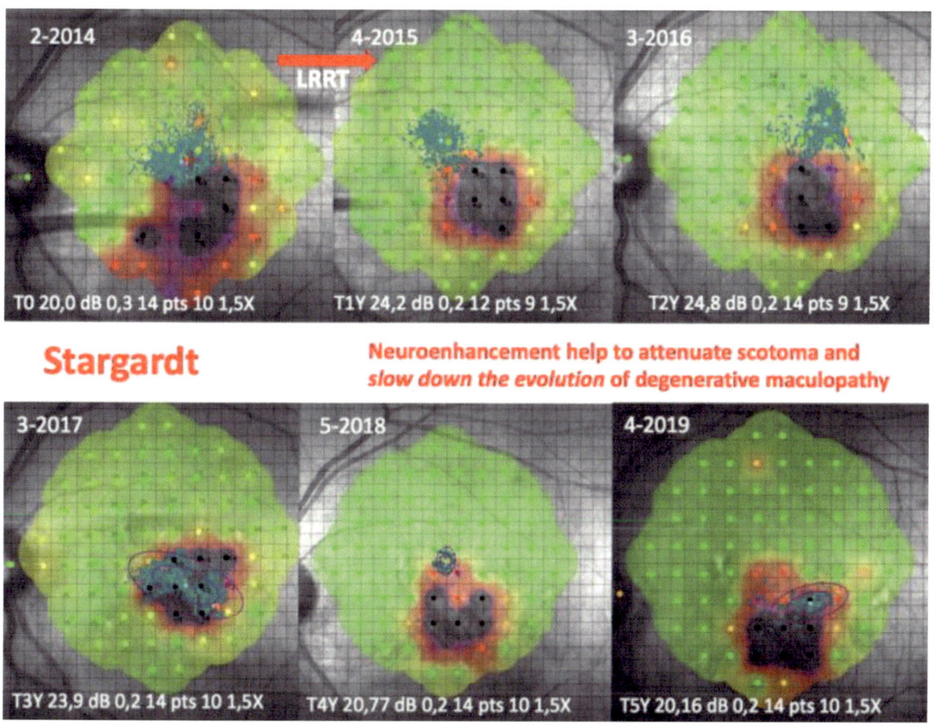

Figure 8.
Patient with molecular diagnosis of Stargardt's maculopathy. In 2014, a suprachoroidal graft of autologous mesenchymal cells was performed. Visual performance after 5 years appears unchanged. Image courtesy of P. Limoli-Milan Low Vision Center.

of this method. We now know for sure that when placed in an appropriate tissue niche stem cells not only survive and proliferate but are capable of differentiating into proper retinal cells which exhibit functional characteristics of real photoreceptors, resulting in the development of a retina-like structure. Further studies are needed to put such promising experimental data into clinical practice and establish standardized procedures for the application of stem cell therapy in the ophthalmological field.

Abbreviations

LESCs	limbal epithelial stem cells
ADSC	adipose-derived stem cells
IPSCs	induced pluripotent stem cells
HPSC	human pluripotent stem cells
MSCs	mesenchymal stem cells
ESCs	embryonic stem cells
TAC	transit amplifying cells
LSCD	limbal stem cell deficiency
ABCG2	ATP-binding cassette family G member 2
CK	cytokeratin
AMD	age-related macular disease
RPE	retinal pigment epithelium
ERG	electroretinography
BCVA	best corrected visual acuity
RGC	retinal ganglion cells
RP	retinitis pigmentosa
DR	diabetic retinopathy
FGF	fibroblast growth factor
VEGF	vascular endothelial growth factor
GM-CSF	granulocyte-macrophage colony stimulating factor
M-CSF	macrophage colony stimulating factor
PIGF	placental growth factor
TGFβ	transforming growth factor beta
HG	hepatocyte growth factor
IGF-1	insulin growth factor
IL	interleukin
CNTF	ciliary neurotrophic factor
BDNF	brain-derived neurotrophic factor
EGF	epidermal growth factor
PEDF	pigmented epithelium-derived factor
PDGF	platelet-derived growth factor
PDAF	platelet-derived angiogenesis factor
TSP	thrombospondin
MC	Muller cells
SOD	superoxide dismutase
IFN-β	interferon beta
IL-1 RA	interleukin 1 receptor antagonist
MCP-1	chemoattractant monocyte protein 1
PGE2R	prostaglandin E2 receptor
CNTF	ciliary neurotrophic factor
ES	electrical stimulation
VP	visual performance

LRRT	Limoli retinal restoration technique
OS	external segment
ASC	adipose stromal cells
PLT	adipose tissue and platelets
PRP	platelet rich plasma

Author details

Enzo Maria Vingolo[1]*, Laura Contento[1], Antonio Florido[1], Filippo Avogaro[1] and Paolo Giuseppe Limoli[2]

1 Department of Medical-Surgical Sciences and Biotechnologies, U.O.C. Ophthalmology, Sapienza University of Rome, Terracina, Italy

2 Low Vision Center, Milan, Italy

*Address all correspondence to: enzomaria.vingolo@uniroma1.it

References

[1] Öner A. Stem cell treatment in retinal diseases: Recent developments. Turkish Journal of Ophthalmology. 2018;**48**(1):33-38

[2] Park SS, Bauer G, Abedi M, Pontow S, Panorgias A, Jonnal R, et al. Intravitreal autologous bone marrow CD34+ cell therapy for ischemic and degenerative retinal disorders: Preliminary phase 1 clinical trial findings. Investigative Ophthalmology & Visual Science. 2015;**56**(1):81-89

[3] Li T, Lewallen M, et al. Multipotent stem cells isolated from the adult mouse retina are capable of producing functional photoreceptors cells. Cell Research. 2013;**23**(6):788-802

[4] Boucherie C, Mukherjee S, Henckaerts E, Thrasher AJ, Sowden JC, Ali RR. Brief report: Self-organizing neuroepithelium from human pluripotent stem cells facilitates derivation of photoreceptors. Stem Cells. 2013;**31**(2):408-414

[5] Schwartz SD, Hubschman JP, Heilwell G, Franco-Cardenas V, et al. Embryonic stem cell trials for macular degeneration: A preliminary report. Lancet. 2012;**379**(9817):713-720

[6] Lu B, Malcuit C, Wang S, Girman S, Francis P, Lemieux L, et al. Long-term safety and function of RPE from human embryonic stem cells in preclinical models of macular degeneration. Stem Cells. 2009;**27**(9):2126-2135

[7] Oswald J, Baranov P. Regenerative medicine in the retina: From stem cells to cell replacement therapy. Therapeutic Advances in Ophthalmology [Internet]. SAGE Publications; January 2018;**10**:1-21. DOI: 10.1177/2515841418774433

[8] Singh R, Cuzzani O, Binette F, Sternberg H, West MD, Nasonkin IO. Pluripotent stem cells for retinal tissue engineering: Current status and future prospects. Stem Cell Reviews and Reports. 2018;**14**(4):463-483

[9] Harvey SU, Pik SC, Franz MC. Stem cell therapy: A novel approach for vision restoration in retinitis pigmentosa. Medical Hypothesis, Discovery & Innovation in Ophthalmology. 2013;**2**(2):52-55

[10] Punzo C, Wenjun X, Cepko Costance L. Loss of Daylight Vision in Retinal Degeneration: Are Oxidative Stress and Metabolic Dysregulation to Blame? Journal of Biological Chemistry [Internet]. American Society for Biochemistry & Molecular Biology (ASBMB); 10 November 2011;287(3):1642-1648. DOI: 10.1074/jbc.r111.304428

[11] Langmann T. Microglia activation in retinal degeneration. Journal of Leukocyte Biology. 2007;**81**:1345-1351

[12] Yafai Y, Iandiev I, Lange J, Yang XM, Wiedemann P, Bringmann A, et al. Basic fibroblast growth factor contributes to a shift in the angioregulatory activity of retinal glial (Müller) cells. PLoS One. 2013;**8**(7):e68773. DOI: 10.1371/journal.pone.0068773

[13] Otani A et al. Rescue of retinal degeneration by intravitreally injected adult bone marrow–derived lineage-negative hematopoietic stem cells. The Journal of Clinical Investigation. 2004;**114**:765-774. DOI: 10.1172/JCI200421686

[14] Guadagni V, Novelli E, Strettoi E. Environmental enrichment reduces photoreceptor degeneration and retinal inflammation in a mouse model of retinitis pigmentosa. Investigative Ophthalmology & Visual Science. 2015;**56**(7):4261-4261

[15] Daftarian N, Kiani S, Zahabi A. Regenerative therapy for retinal

disorders. Journal of Ophthalmic and Vision Research. 2010;**5**:250-264

[16] Jones MK, Lu B, Girman S, Wang S. Cell-based therapeutic strategies for replacement and preservation in retinal degenerative diseases. Progress in Retinal and Eye Research [Internet]. Elsevier BV; May 2017;**58**:1-27. DOI: 10.1016/j.preteyeres.2017.01.004

[17] Ding SLS, Kumar S, Mok PL. Cellular reparative mechanisms of mesenchymal stem cells for retinal diseases. International Journal of Molecular Sciences. 2017;**18**:1406

[18] Dominici M, Le Blanc K, Mueller I, et al. Minimal criteria for defining multipotent mesenchymal stromal cells. The International Society for Cellular Therapy position statement. Cytotherapy. 2006;**8**(4):315-317

[19] Baddour JA, Sousounis K, Tsonis PA. Organ repair and regeneration: An overview. Birth Defects Research C: Embryo Today. 2012;**96**(1):1-29. DOI: 10.1002/bdrc.21006

[20] Zarbin M. Cell-based therapy for degenerative retinal disease. Trends in Molecular Medicine. 2016;**22**:115-134. DOI: 10.1016/j.molmed.2015.12.007

[21] Konno M, Hamabe A, Hasegawa S, Ogawa H, Fukusumi T, Nishikawa S, et al. Adipose-derived mesenchymal stem cells and regenerative medicine. Development, Growth & Differentiation. 2013;**55**:309-318. DOI: 10.1111/dgd.12049

[22] Rezanejad H, Soheili ZS, Haddad F, Matin MM, Samiei S, Manafi A, et al. In vitro differentiation of adipose-tissue-derived mesenchymal stem cells into neural retinal cells through expression of human PAX6 (5a) gene. Cell and Tissue Research. 2014;**356**:65-75. DOI: 10.1007/s00441-014-1795-y

[23] Anitua E, Andia I, Ardanza B, Nurden P, Nurden AT. Autologous platelets as a source of proteins for healing and tissue regeneration. Thrombosis and Haemostasis. 2004;**91**(1):4-15

[24] Wahlin KJ, Campochiaro PA, Zack DJ, Adler R. Neurotrophic factors cause activation of intracellular signaling pathways in Muller cells and other cells of the inner retina, but not photoreceptors. Investigative Ophthalmology and Visual Science. 2000;**41**:927-936

[25] Frasson M, Picaud S, Leveillard T, Simonutti M, Mohand-Said S, Dreyfus H, et al. Glial cell line-derived neurotrophic factor induces histologic and functional protection of rod photoreceptors in the rd/rd mouse. Investigative Ophthalmology and Visual Science. 1999;**40**:2724-2734

[26] Limoli PG, Vingolo EM, Morales MU, Nebbioso M, Limoli C. Preliminary study on electrophysiological changes after cellular autograft in age-related macular degeneration. Medicine. 2014;**93**(29):e355. DOI: 10.1097/MD.0000000000000355

[27] Limoli PG, Vingolo EM, Limoli C, Scalinci SZ, Nebbioso M. Regenerative therapy by suprachoroidal cell autograft in dry age-related macular degeneration: Preliminary in vivo report. Journal of Visualized Experiments. 2018;**132**. DOI: 10.3791/56469

[28] Mammoto T, Jiang A, Jiang E, Mammoto A. Platelet rich plasma extract promotes angiogenesis through the angiopoietin1-Tie2 pathway. Microvascular Research. 2013;**89**:15-24. DOI: 10.1016/j.mvr.2013.04.008

[29] Sheibani N, Sorenson CM, Cornelius LA, et al. Thrombospondin-1, a natural inhibitor of angiogenesis, is present in vitreous and aqueous humor and is modulated by hyperglycemia.

Biochemical and Biophysical Research Communications. 2000;**267**:257-261

[30] Lieberthal W, Triaca V, Koh JS, Pagano PJ, Levine JS. Role of superoxide in apoptosis induced by growth factor withdrawal. The American Journal of Physiology. 1998;**275**(5 Pt 2):F691-F702

[31] Yu DY, Cringle SJ. Retinal degeneration and local oxygen metabolism. Experimental Eye Research. 2005;**80**(6):745-751

[32] Yamada H, Yamada E, Ando A, et al. Fibroblast growth factor-2 decreases hyperoxia-induced photoreceptor cell death in mice. American Journal of Pathology. 2001;**159**(3):1113-1120

[33] Cui Y, Xu N, Xu W, Xu G. Mesenchymal stem cells attenuate hydrogen peroxide-induced oxidative stress and enhance neuroprotective effects in retinal ganglion cells. In Vitro Cellular & Developmental Biology: Animal. 2016;**53**:328-335

[34] Zeng HY, Zhu XA, Zhang C, Yang LP, Wu LM, Tso MOM. Identification of sequential events and factors associated with microglial activation, migration, and cytotoxicity in retinal degeneration in rd mice. Investigative Ophthalmology & Visual Science. 2005;**46**(8):2992-2999

[35] Peng B, Xiao J, Wang K, So K-F, Tipoe GL, Lin B. Suppression of microglial activation is neuroprotective in a mouse model of human retinitis pigmentosa. The Journal of Neuroscience. 2014;**34**(24):8139-8150

[36] Bakondi B, Girman S, Lu B, Wang S. Multimodal delivery of isogenic mesenchymal stem cells yields synergistic protection from retinal degeneration and vision loss. Stem Cells Translational Medicine. 2017;**6**:444-457

[37] Schneider A, Krüger C, Steigleder T, et al. The hematopoietic factor G-CSF is a neuronal ligand that counteracts programmed cell death and drives neurogenesis. The Journal of Clinical Investigation. 2005;**115**:2083-2098

[38] Athanasiou D, Aguilà M, Bevilacqua D, Novoselov SS, Parfitt DA, Cheetham ME. The cell stress machinery and retinal degeneration. FEBS Letters. 2013;**587**:2008-2017

[39] Kim SY, Mocanu C, McLeod DS, et al. Expression of pigment epithelium-derived factor (PEDF) and vascular endothelial growth factor (VEGF) in sickle cell retina and choroid. Experimental Eye Research. 2003;**77**:433-445

[40] Zack DJ. Neurotrophic rescue of photoreceptors: are Müller cells the mediators of survival? Neuron. 2000;**26**:285-286

[41] Atashi F, Jaconi ME, Pittet-Cuénod B, Modarressi A. Autologous platelet-rich plasma: A biological supplement to enhance adipose-derived mesenchymal stem cell expansion. Tissue Engineering Part C: Methods. 2015;**21**(3):253-262. DOI: 10.1089/ten.TEC.2014.0206

[42] LaVail MM, Faktorovich EG, Hepler JM, et al. Basic fibroblast growth factor protects photoreceptors from light-induced degeneration in albino rats. Annals of the New York Academy of Sciences. 1991;**638**:341-347

[43] Manthey AL, Liu W, Jiang ZX, Lee MHK, Ji J, So KF, et al. Using electrical stimulation to enhance the efficacy of cell transplantation therapies for neurodegenerative retinal diseases: Concepts, challenges, and future perspectives. Cell Transplantation. 2017;**26**(6):949-965. DOI: 10.3727/096368917X694877

[44] Ciavatta VT, Kim M, Wong P, Nickerson JM, Shuler RK Jr, McLean GY, et al. Retinal expression of Fgf2 in RCS rats with subretinal microphotodiode

array. Investigative Ophthalmology and Visual Science. 2009;**50**:4523-4530

[45] Schmid H, Herrmann T, Kohler K, Stett A. Neuroprotective effect of transretinal electrical stimulation on neurons in the inner nuclear layer of the degenerated retina. Brain Research Bulletin. 2009;**79**:15-25

[46] Oner A, Sevim DG. Complications of stem cell based therapies in retinal diseases. Stem Cell Research Open Library. 2017;**1**(1):1-7

[47] Lawrence N, Coleman WP. Liposuction. Journal of the American Academy of Dermatology. 2002;**47**:105-108

[48] Kevy SV et al. Preparation of growth factor enriched autologous platelet gel. In: Transactions of the Society for Biomaterials 27th Annual Meeting. St. Paul, Minnesota, USA, April 24-29. 2001

[49] Tischler M. Platelet rich plasma: The use of autologous growth factors to enhance bone and soft tissue grafts. The New York State Dental Journal. 2002;**68**:22

[50] Oner A, Gonen ZB, Sevim DG, Sinim Kahraman N, Unlu M. Six-month results of suprachoroidal adipose tissue-derived mesenchymal stem cell implantation in patients with optic atrophy: A phase 1/2 study. International Ophthalmology [Internet]. Springer Science and Business Media LLC; 15 July 2019;**39**(12):2913-2922. DOI: 10.1007/ s10792 019 01141 5

[51] Limoli P. The retinal cell-neuroregeneration. Principles, applications and perspectives. In: Limoli Retina Regeneration Technique [Italian]. San Giovanni 40, Canelli (AT): FGE Reg.; 2014. pp. 407-424

Chapter 5

Application of Nanowires for Retinal Regeneration

Davood Kharaghani, Zahra Tajbakhsh, Phan Duy Nam and Ick Soo Kim

Abstract

Nanowires aim at developing advanced architectures are gaining popularity for damaged neural systems. The retina with a complicated structure is an essential part of our visual nervous system. Any disorder inside retina could lead to blindness due to irregularity in transferring neural signals to the brain. In recent years, the emergence of nanostructures, as well as nanowires, has provided a viable means for enhancing the regeneration of retinal. Nanowires with the ability to sense light and converting it to the electrical signals simulate the extracellular electrical properties, which are the newest nanostructures for the retinal applications. The different structure of nanowires has been examined in vitro, and several others are undergoing in vivo for vision recovery. Among the structures, core-shell nanowires and functionalized nanowires with gold nanoparticles attract the attention for the regeneration of retinal neural systems. Herein, subsequently provide an introduction to the anatomy of the retina, and retinal disorders, the latest progress in the regeneration of retina and vision using nanowires will be reviewed. Also, the different structures, including core-shell and functionalized nanowires with nanoparticles, will be examined. Eventually, the point of view and perspective of applying nanowire in retinal regeneration will be offered.

Keywords: regeneration of retina, nanowires in ophthalmology, nanowires for tissue engineering, nanowires biocompatibility

1. Introduction

The retinal transplantation is limited due to the complex neural network [1]. Retina senses light and converts it into the neural signals and transfers neural signals to the brain and cause visual perception [2, 3]. Nanostructures have evolved as multidisciplinary applications by combination with materials as an advanced architecture to develop functional substitutes for various proposes such as wound dressing [4–6], tissue engineering [7–11], and biomedical applications [12–14]. Neuroscience, related to the retina is one of the most exciting fields where nanostructures with modified properties serve as scaffolds to promote and facilitate the migration and adhesion of the cells [15].

Until recently, it was believed that scaffolds simulated the extracellular matrix (EMC) in the regeneration of retina, and served as a support for cell migration, adhesion, and morphology only [16–18]. Emphasis was on loaded materials and morphology construction to develop biocompatible and biodegradable scaffolds with appropriate mechanical properties [19–22]. However, the first definition of tissue regeneration is developing scaffolds with acceptable biocompatibility to implant in the host body to repair damaged tissues or organs. Therefore, the electrospun nanofibers with a high ratio of surface-to-volume, tunable porosity, and similarity to natural EMC show the ability to modify the surface functions with different structures for a wide range of tissue regeneration [23]. Nanofibers have emerged as a potential to simulate the ECM in many tissues such as bone [10], nerves [24], and various techniques have been employed to fabricate the nanofibers with excellent properties [25].

As extracellular electrical simulation involves in neuroscience and neural tissue engineering [26–28], attention is focused on nanowires applications for visual neural system [29–31], brain [32, 33] and cardiac [34]. Nanowires have recognized as widely used nanostructure for the cell microenvironment where the electrodynamic properties [35] have permanently affected cellular functions, such as morphology, adhesion, differentiation, and proliferation [36]. As a consequence, researchers have developed new structures for better electroconductivity, biocompatibility, and cell adhesion [37–39].

Nanowires have been shown that simulate the nerve signals in the retina and transfer between the layers could improve the vision loss by the damaged retina. To explain the recovery of vision with nanowires, which lost by retinal degeneration, we will begin by describing the retinal anatomy, and how various retinal disorders may cause blindness. Then we will investigate the nanowires which could enhance retinal organization with sensing light and converting it to the electrochemical signals with different materials, structures, and properties. Finally, we will discuss the challenges ahead and prospect in the application of nanowires for recovery of vision that lost by retinal destruction.

2. Retina

2.1 Anatomy of the retina

The retina is the innermost multilayered structure of the eye with an approximate thickness of 0.50 mm [40]. Retina first translates light into a biochemical message and then prepared biochemical messages converted into the electrical messages, cause to the visual information with transmitted to the primary visual cortex of the brain via the optic nerve.

The retina is composed of retinal pigment epithelium (RPE) and neuroretina, which is further divided into nine layers. Respectively, the neuroretina layer includes the outer and inner segments of photoreceptors (PL), outer limiting membrane, outer nuclear layer (ONL), outer plexiform layer (OPL), inner nuclear layer [41], inner plexiform layer (IPL), ganglion cell layer (GCL), nerve fiber layer (NFL) and inner limiting membrane (ILM) from nearest layer to choroid up to nearest layer to vitreous [40]. This part is consists of five types of neurons: the visual receptors cells (the rods and cones), the horizontal cells, the bipolar cells, the amacrine cells, and the retinal ganglion cells [42].

RPE with a function to absorb light is a monolayer of pigmented hexagonal cells which are denser in the macular area. Mostly, the interaction between RPE and photoreceptors has a significant effect on the ability of photoreceptors to detect light and convert the light into the electrical signals, which caused vision preparation [43]. RPE is separated from the choroid by the Bruch's membrane. As RPE is located between the outer segments of the photoreceptors and the vascular layer of the choroid, it has a two-directional function. RPE with transports ions, water, and metabolic products from the subretinal space to the blood and receiving nutrients such as glucose and retinol from the blood to nourish the photoreceptors playing the critical role in the retina layer. However, failure in mentioned functions can lead to retinal degeneration, visual loss, and eventually blindness [43].

PL is the only light-sensitive part of the neuroretina and is composed of outer and inner segments of the rod and cone cells. Cone cells are responsible for color detection and are found in high number in the macula, especially foveal region, whereas rods are more active in the dark and are abundant in the peripheral retina. OLM layer separates PL from the photoreceptor nuclei, and it is not considered as an actual layer. ONL contains the nuclei of photoreceptors, and its thickness varies across the retina with the maximum thickness at the fovea. However, the axons of the photoreceptors cells and their synapses with bipolar and horizontal cells form the OPL. On the other hand, cell bodies of horizontal cells, bipolar cells, amacrine cells, and Muller glial cells are in the INL layer. The INL layer, playing the critical role to transmit inputs signals from IPL to OPL, which is composed of synapses between the bipolar, ganglion, and amacrine cells. The innermost layer of the retina is GCL and located in the place near to the vitreous and contains the cell bodies of ganglion cells and displaced amacrine cells, astrocytes, and Muller cell bodies that their axons converge on the way to the optic disc and form NFL. The latest layer of the retina is ILM, which forms the inner boundary of the retina on the vitreous side. **Figure 1** is showing the retinal layer that divided into nine layers with nine different cell type [40].

The macula is a region inside the retina which contains the highest number of ganglion cells and cause the optimal vision and color perception process [44]. Rods and cones are responsible for the initiation of the scotopic and photopic visual processing, respectively. When the light absorbed by photoreceptors, rod, and cone cells with releasing glutamate as a neurotransmitter cause to transfer the electrical signals from synapse onto the bipolar cells at the OPL layer. Afterward, transferring

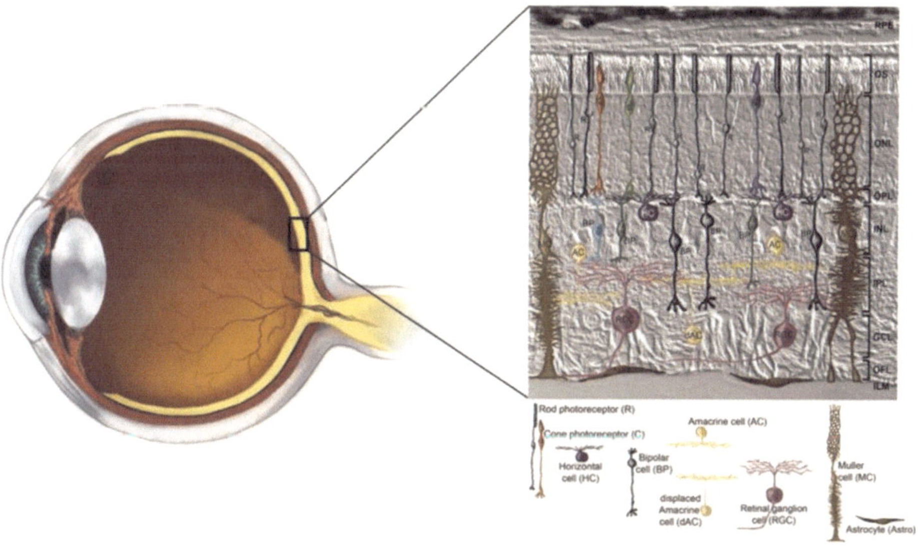

Figure 1.
The anatomy of retina from outer layer (up) to inner layer (down) is containing of retinal pigment epithelium (RPE), outer segment of photoreceptors (OS), outer nuclear layer (ONL), outer plexiform layer (OPL), inner nuclear layer [41], inner plexiform layer (IPL), ganglion cell layer (GCL), inner segments of photoreceptors (IPL), optic fiber layer (OFL), and inner limiting membrane (ILM) from nearest to choroid to nearest to vitreous, respectively. The retina is consist of nine cell line consisting of rod photoreceptor (R), cone photoreceptors (C), horizontal cells (HC), bipolar cells (BC), amacrine cells (AC), displaced amacrine cells (dAC), retinal ganglion cells (RGC), Muller cells, and astrocyte cells (Astro) [2].

the electrical signals from bipolar cells synapse by amacrine and ganglion cells at the IPL to the axons of the ganglion cells lead to the output neurons signals formation as the optic nerve and deliver the visual information to the brain [45].

2.2 Retinal pathology

It is reported that half of the blindness in the world is related to the various retinal damages. Degenerative damages such as age-related macular degeneration (AMD) and retinitis pigmentosa (RP), optic neuropathy such as glaucoma and vascular retinopathy as well as diabetic retinopathy (DR) are the most common retinal diseases and the leading causes of legal blindness [46].

AMD is an age-related retinal problem occur in two forms of dry and wet. The dry form is mainly diagnosed by drusen and extracellular materials deposition such as lipids and proteins which accumulate in Bruch's membrane, and loss of photoreceptors by geographic atrophy of the macula. However, wet form or neovascular/exudative AMD is diagnosed by choroidal neovascularization (CNV), blood vessel development and hemorrhage/leakage of blood and fluid accumulation into the neural retina which can lead to the RPE detachment. The hallmark of AMD is the degeneration of neurons in the macula, which may result in central vision loss at the early stage of the disease [47].

RP refers as a hereditary and neurodegenerative disease of the retina may appear in different forms. The outcome in all forms is photoreceptor degeneration and subsequently, cell death. Photoreceptor degeneration starts from the periphery of the retina, which progressively decreases the visual field and consequently makes a tunnel vision for the patient. Vision impairments in RP will start with rod photoreceptors and followed by cone photoreceptors degeneration that latter can lead to alteration and abnormalities in the RPE [48].

Glaucoma is the most common optic nerve disease that can lead to blindness. Glaucoma with increasing the intraocular pressure may cause retinal ganglion cells degeneration. However, disorders in the retinal nerve fiber layer and optic nerve proceed during glaucoma and will lead to irreversible vision loss if the treatment is not appropriate [49].

DR as vascular retinopathy is another cause for blindness in the worldwide which divided into type-one and type-two. There is evidence for possible dysfunction of Muller cell during diabetic neuropathy [50]. DR is classified into the proliferative stage with loss of blood supply and non-proliferative stage with altered retinal vascular permeability, intraretinal microaneurysms, and macular edema [51].

There is no definite cure for retinal diseases, and most of them end up with severe visual impairment or blindness. Current medical treatments may help to decrease the progression of the disease and are unable to cure them. Therefore there is a need for novel approaches to target restoring partial vision by preparing the advanced structure as well as nanowires and nanomedicines.

3. Structure and overview of nanowires

Nanostructures could be useful to follow the development of advanced structures for retinal applications where functionality depends on materials properties. Moreover, the combination of scaffolds with existing nanomaterials may improve the required functions [52]. In a recent study, nanowires with various structures have been used for regeneration of retina. The synthesis and fabrication of nanowires, with a narrow range of subtracting such as gold and TiO_2 nanoparticles combined with polymers as well as poly (e-caprolactone) cast onto anodized aluminum oxide template, have been used for retinal regeneration applications [53–55].

Gallium phosphide is another example of materials have been employed for the regeneration of retinal. Gallium phosphide as multimodel nanowire employed for different geometries such as rod and cone photoreceptor, ganglion cells, and bipolar cells [56]. Also, the same structure coated with poly-L-ornithine showed that nanowires have significant potential on morphology, adhesion, and metabolism of cells in comparison to the flat surface [57, 58].

The nanostructures designs based on silicone, to simulate the retina photoreceptor was improved by nanomaterials coating as well as gold and titanium oxide nanoparticles [59]. Whereas, silicon nanowires have been shown to form spontaneous conjunction with photoreceptor cells. Such nanostructures showed that they could improve the quality of photoreceptor simulation and increase cell adhesion to the nanowires when placed in direct contact with cells [60].

Silicon nanowires coated with gold were shown to be more effective at the simulation of photoreceptors; this is mostly attributed to the higher surface to the area for sensing light and charge transfer [61, 62]. Another type of nanostructures is thin films functionalized with the nanoparticle to sense light. Thine film structures were able to simulate cultured photoreceptors when subjected to direct visible light [50, 63–65].

In addition to sense light, nanowires can use for transferring the electrical signals through the cells such as rode and cone cells [66]. One way for transfer signals between the nanostructures and cells is to simulate solar panels structure in nanosize via materials such as *n-type* and *p-type* silicon, which can sense the light and convert the light signals into the electrical signals. In particular, silicon nanowires are useful to sense light and transfer the signals to the internal layer of the retina to recover the eyesight [67, 68].

The architecture of nanowires has been clarified as complex core-shell nanowires with complex chemical profiles. These advanced structures have been

Nanowire	Forms	Length (μm)	Modification	Refs
Iridium wire	Pillar array electrode	75	Embedded with glass	[66]
Poly (e-caprolactone)	Nanowire	2.5–27.5	Cast onto anodized aluminum oxide template	[53]
Poly (e-caprolactone)	Short nanowire	2.5	Electrospinning method	[55]
Gallium phosphide	Nanowire	0.5–4	Gold nanoparticles	[56]
Parylene/silicon	Silicon tip	Not reported	Platinum and gold tine film	[59]
Gallium phosphide	Functionalized nanowire	Not reported	Gold/palladium nanoparticles, nanowires coated with poly-L-ornithine	[57]
Silicon	Nanowire/ microelectrode	20	Coated by polyimide	[62]
n-type silicon	Nanowire	Not reported	Gold/palladium nanoparticles	[60]
Titanium dioxide	Nanowire	Not reported	Gold nanoparticles	[67]
n-type/*p-type* silicon	Coaxial nanowire	Not reported	Gold nanoparticles	[69]

Table 1.
The materials have been used to prepare the nanowires structure for retinal implant applications.

made from *n-type* and *p-type* silicon for making connections between the membranes of live bipolar cells and nanowires to sense the light for the recovery of vision [69]. **Table 1** represents the materials have been used as nanowires for vision recovery lost due to retinal disorders.

4. Nanowire based mechanism of retina regeneration

4.1 Extracellular matrix simulation and cell adhesion

Tissue engineering specified as two foremost policies to redevelop the injured tissues or organs such as (1) cell-based; when cells are the critical substance to modify the place before transplanted to the host body, and (2) scaffold-based; when an extracellular matrix (ECM) from biomaterials designed and simulate in vivo structures. Recreating the retina requires effective architecture to mimic the extracellular matrix with physiological and morphological features resembling the in vivo structure [70]. The ECM with the composition of an intricate interweaving of protein provides the appropriate structure for cells grow with vast morphogenesis, which creates the vary forms of tissue and organs. However, the ECM classified into the two main categories of interstitial and pericellular. The interstitial matrices define as matrices that surround cells, whereas; pericellular matrices are with close contact with cells. The obvious example is the basement membrane, which is a type of pericellular matrix, and with providing an anchoring, membrane prevents parenchymal cells to break apart [71]. Also, unique ECM is associate to differentiate, changes in morphology and topography of cells to form the unique tissue and organs [72].

The mature mammalian retina is consists of two basement layer such as Brunch membrane at the interface between retinal pigment epithelium (RPE) membrane and choroid and second is the inner limiting membrane (ILM) at the interface of the neural retina with the vitreous body [73]. **Figure 2** is showing the two basement layers in the structure of the retina and their morphogenesis.

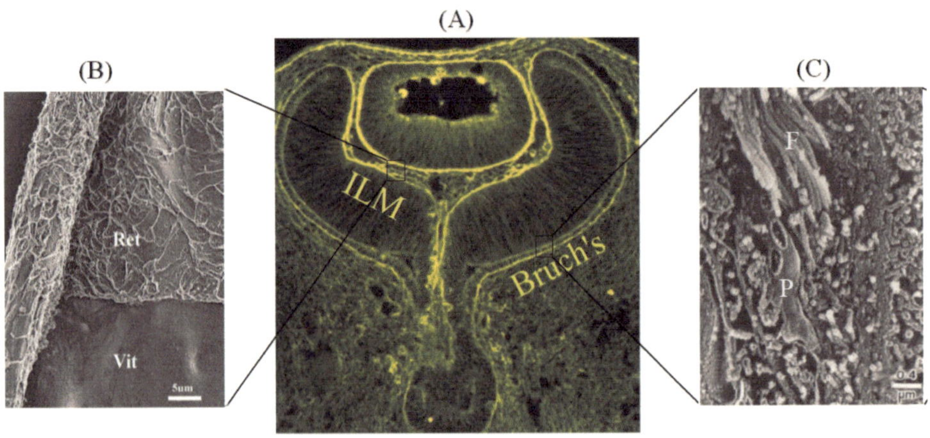

Figure 2.
Immunohistochemistry of the 8 weeks gestation human that stained with the immunofluorescent antibody. The yellow line labeled are showing the Bruch's and ILM membrane that continues the same identical membrane folded over inside the eye (A), the scanning electron microscope of the ILM membrane showing that the surface in contact with RPE (Ret) is irregular whereas the vitread surface (Vit) represents the smooth surface (B), and Bruch's membrane showing the composition of aligned collagenous fibers (F) in composition of cell process (C) [74, 75].

Recently, Kharaghani and co-workers [76] reported a study emphasizing the importance of morphogenesis in the three-dimension (3D) nanofibers scaffold structure in guiding the seeded cells for ophthalmic tissue engineering mainly for cornea and retinal applications. The necessities for using scaffolds in ophthalmic tissue engineering are cell adhesion besides to tensile strength, effectiveness on cell morphology, and topography of scaffolds [76]. This report stressed the significance of the underlying ECM in endorsing exclusive micro and nanoenvironments that fosters tissue regeneration. However, it is unfortunate that there is no report about the study of ECM simulation by nanowires or surface chemistry of nanowires that shows cell adhesion, where it is used for retinal regeneration. At the moment, all reports have been used the single nanowire for the regeneration of retina.

In attempts to control the cell adhesion on nanowires, researchers repopulated their strategy to change the surface chemistry nanowires prepared based on titanium, silicon, and zinc [77–79]. However, the in vitro and in vivo researches have been don around the regeneration of retina by nanowires, and results show that cells tended to encompass. Also, it should be happening due to electrical stimulation of place based on the extracellular electrical.

4.2 Extracellular electrical simulation

It is mentioned here earlier that converts light into the neural signals and transfer neural signals to the brain by retina will lead to visual perception. Extracellular electrical involving ion channels has a vital role in nervous systems such as the retina. Photovoltaic polymers such as silk have been shown the great potential to use a connection between the layer of the retina to restore the vision with transfer the electrical signals [80]. The intracellular voltage is one of the unknown metrics that many types of research have been focused on recording signal strength use a nanoscale electrode as well as nanowires. Nanowires have been shown the tremendous potential upon extracellular electrical stimulation of cells to promote cell growth, adhesion, and differentiation. Also, Vodovnik and coworkers showed that the external electrical field had a significant effect on the polarization of cells on the cathodal and anodal side of the electrode [81].

On the other hand, the positive and negative charge should be optimized for the clinical implant to achieve successful results. The cationic polymers and nanoparticles with high concentrations of nitrogen may help to compaction of negative charge DNA and RNA and lead to better gens protection and endosomal escape in addition to high transaction efficiency and stability [2]. **Figure 3** is showing how nanowires with simulating the extracellular electric could cause cell adhesion to the nanowires and effect on the recovery of vision after implantation in mice eye.

Among the various nanostructures, gold nanoparticles due to high electroconductivity, biocompatibility, and chemical inertness have been attracting the attention to develop scaffolds for neural systems such as retinal applications. However, it is unfortunate that the development of high-quality gold nanowires faces challenges in the absence of robust methods for synthesis. Nevertheless, the gold nanoparticle with the electrical resistance of 52 Ω is one of inseparable part of scaffolds have been used for retinal applications as reported in **Table 1**, which gold nanoparticles have embedded with nanowire structures [61].

In an attempt to design an implantable electronic device for regeneration of retina when photoreceptors are damaged, electrically stimulate of retinal neurons, become an essential challenge. Whereas, several retinal prostheses are going on, but none of them have shown the ability to evoke phosphenes in blindness. Refer to retinal anatomy controlling the signal impedance is the most crucial subject to

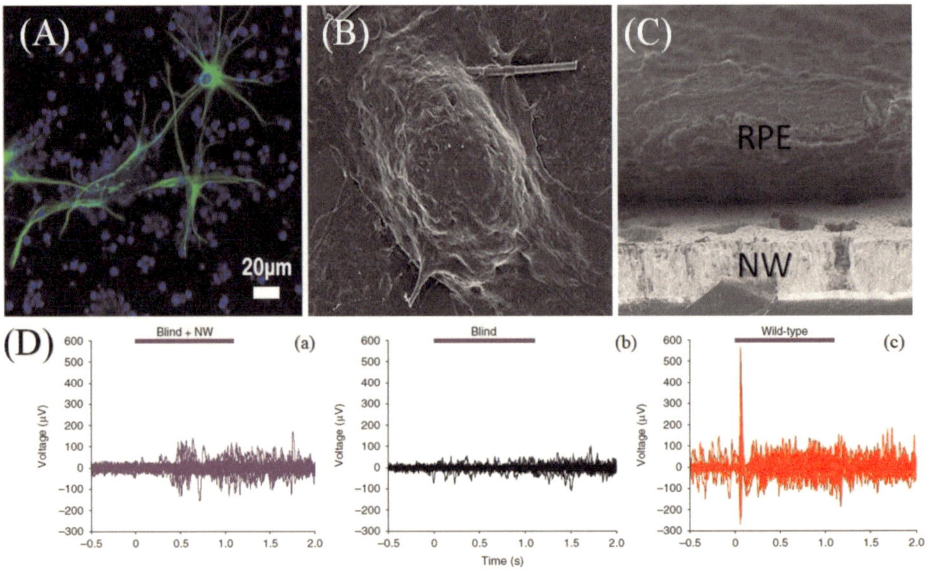

Figure 3.
The immunohistochemical graph of glial cells from mouse have been cultured on gallium nanowires, the cells stained green by glial fibrillary acidic protein (GFAP) and cells nuclei stained blue by 4,6-diamidino-2-phenylindole (DAPI) (A), SEM image from rat dorsal root ganglion cell surrounded a single a coaxial n-type/p-type *silicon nanowire (B), SEM image from interface between the mice retina (RPE) and titanium dioxide array nanowire modified by gold nanoparticles (C), and the response of UV-light-evoked in the blind mice retina after implantation with titanium dioxide array nanowires modified with gold nanoparticles (a), blind mice without any implantation (b) and control (c) [67, 69, 82].*

prepare the appropriate prosthesis due to discerption of the retina as a layered structure with different electrical conductivity for each layer which the inner layers have higher resistivity in comparison to outer layers such as retinal epithelial pigment and membrane [83].

However, among the different research, simulation of photovoltaic materials, as well as silicon and titanium nanowires functionalized by gold nanoparticles that have the ability to receive the light signals and change the light signals to the electrical signals, are attracting the interests [68, 84]. Also, photovoltaic nanowires started the new generation of materials with extracellular electrical simulation and conjunction with the cells that are remaining the main challenges as implants used for retinal regeneration (**Table 2**).

4.3 Light sensation

Nanowires have been explored extensively as a component of photovoltaic to improve the efficiency of sensing light for retinal applications. The use of single nanowire as photovoltaic nanostructures present the several crucial advantages, which may leverage to produce robust, high efficiency and compatibility with cells. The simple example of sensing light and converting the light signals to the electrical signals are solar cells made from *n-type* and *p-type* silicon. Briefly, the *p-type* silicon produced by materials that have one free place for accepting one extra electron on the outer layer of orbital despite the *n-type* silicone which produced by elements and has one extra electron in the outer layer of their orbital and electron is not involved in any bonding. However, light absorption by the *n-type* silicon layer will cause to the movement of an extra electron to the empty orbital of *p-type* silicon, and this electron movement between the *n-type* and *p-type* silicon layers lead to changing the

Nanowire	In vitro	In vivo	Cell responses	Refs
Iridium wire	—	Subretinal (rat)	Implant connected to inner nuclear layer	[66]
Poly (e-caprolactone)	Retinal progenitor cells	—	Cells developed on the place that short nanowires aggregated	[53]
Poly (e-caprolactone)	—	Subretinal (pigs)	Short nanowires have done better interaction with cells in comparison to electrospun nanofibers.	[55]
Gallium phosphide	Rod and cone photoreceptor, ganglion cells and bipolar cells	—	Glial cell did not overgrow the neurons may be due to topographical of nanowires.	[56]
Parylene/ silicon	—	—		[59]
Gallium phosphide	Cortical neural stem cells	—	Nanowires embedded with cells strongly and nanowires did not have a significant effect on the morphology and RNA microarray	[57]
Silicon	—	—		[62]
n-type silicon	Mice retinal cell	—	The nanowires showed good cell distributions even though the nanowires do not permit the neural network formation.	[60]
Titanium dioxide	—	Subretinal mice	Array nanowires could transfer the neural signals and partly recover the vision of blind mice.	[67]
n-type/p-type silicon	Dorsal root ganglion	—	Cells successfully surrounded the nanowires, and in vitro light senses showed the ability of produced nanowires for senses the light and neural signal transfer.	[69]

Table 2.
The in vitro and in vivo responses of nanowires.

light signals to the electrical signals [41, 85]. **Figure 4** is showing the process of turning light signals to the electrical signals used for regeneration of retinal photoreceptor. Also, sensing the light and electron travels between the *n-type*, *p-type* silicon will cause to the preparation of local extracellular electrical simulation, and conjunction between nanowires and cells as explained earlier. However, the gold nanoparticles with one free electron in the outermost layer of orbital play a vital role in improving the sensitivity of light perception in composition whit coaxial silicon nanowires [86]. Therefore in most of the nanowires have been produced for the regeneration of retina, gold nanoparticles loaded on the surface of nanowires.

Another example of using the same construction introduced by Tang et al. [67] use titanium dioxide nanowire loaded by gold nanoparticles. Also, they show that titanium dioxide nanowire loaded by gold nanoparticles with size 10 nm have the ability to efficient electron injection into the nanowires and implant as photoreceptor simulation in the rat retina success upon photo-illumination [67].

In the past years, nanowires with various structures but the same proposition for the regeneration of retina, recovery of vision have been developed, and their performance has been investigated. The researchers found that nanowires loaded with gold nanoparticles, showed a robust potential compare with cheapest and devices

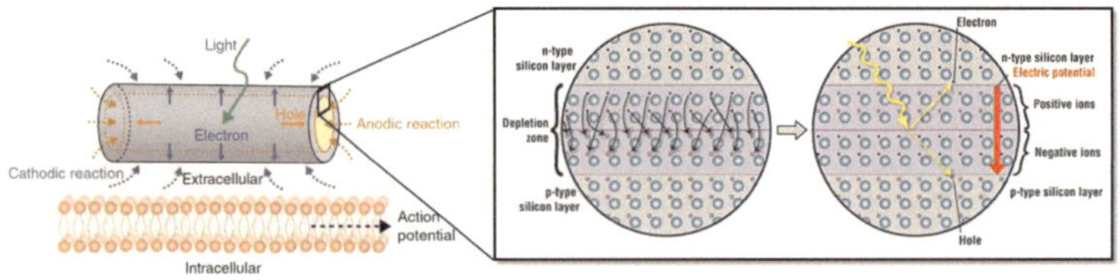

Figure 4.
Schematic of electron movement and holes toward the n-type and p-type silicon at the neural cell membrane for simulating the light senses. Light with receive to the n-type silicon containing the positive ions causes to the movement of electrons to the p-type silicon layer containing negative ions cause to senses the light and transfer produced faradic current to the cells [69]. (Refer to ACS ChemMatters online archive 2013–2014).

for vision recovery lost due to retinal degeneration. Such observation emphasizes that nanowires are starting point in the progress for regeneration and implantable artificial photoreceptors.

5. Challenges and prospects

We believe that future strategies could involve incorporating smart nanostructures to simulate the extracellular matrix in addition to extracellular electric based on the intracellular electric charges to follow the polarization and adhesion of cells in the retina. For example, when the level of light changes, the system would control the transferred electrical signals by implants. Therefore we believe that nanostructures such as carbon nanotubes could serve to control the extracellular electrical charge incorporation nanoparticles such as gold nanoparticles for light sensation with a size of less than 10 nm to control the thermal stability. **Figure 5** is showing the retinal cell polarization when external electrical charge

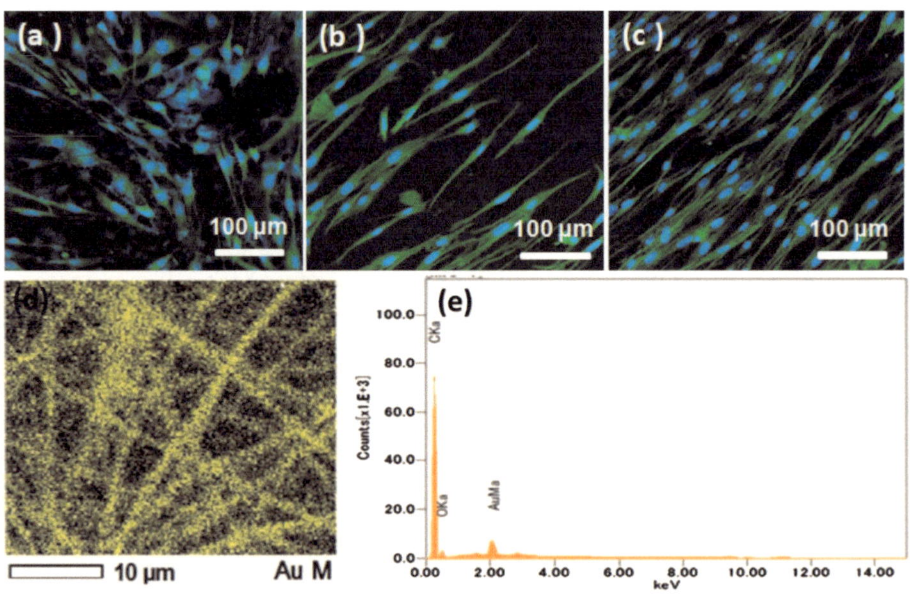

Figure 5.
The confocal microscopy image of seeded retinal ganglion cells into the random polypyrrole/graphene/poly (lactic-co-glycolic acid) nanofibers (a), polypyrrole/graphene nanofibers (b), the aligned polypyrrole/graphene/poly (lactic-co-glycolic acid) nanofibers (c), the SEM mapping of loaded gold nanoparticles into the polyvinylpyrrolidone nanofiber (d) and the energy-dispersive X-ray for loaded gold nanoparticles into the polyvinylpyrrolidone nanofibers (e) [24, 26].

supplied into the aligned nanofiber [26] and how nanofibers can simulate the extracellular matrixwith loading the gold nanoparticles into the nanofibers which done by our team [24].

Finally, we envisage the use of stem cells incorporation of smart nanostructures and instruct the formation and regeneration of retina. Smart nanostructures with the ability to control the neural signals and simulation of the extracellular matrix could potentially circulate inside the retina and repair by cell adhesion, and in conjunction with smart nanostructures followed by transferring the adjusted signals to the brain in order to form clear vision. Therefore, our team has suggested to use the carbon nanowires to prepare the appropriate scaffold that can support both extracellular matrix and extracellular electric for improving the cell adhesion and light sensation.

6. Conclusion

Nanowires have had a substantial impact on retinal applications and still, have great potential to advance therapeutic implants for retinal regeneration. The development of new structures, and their incorporation into the simulation of the extracellular matrix, extracellular electric and light senses may lead to improvement of advanced structure for developing artificial retina. However, challenges still need to be addressed in controlling the local charges and light sensation improvement. It is believed that engineered nanowires with high efficiency will be increasingly used in retinal implantations. In recent years, several in vitro and in vivo reports have indicated the possibility of a significant effect of nanowires on the recovery of vision that lost due to retinal degeneration. Another challenge that must be addressed is the extracellular matrix to create a 3D scaffold, where it did not discuss in reports that have been done for nanowires usage in vision recovery, due to a limitation in synthesizing of nanowires. Also, it is crucial to discover the key factor promoting the assemblies of different layers of the retina and create specific scaffolds for polarization and construction of cells for transferring the neural signals to the brain. Developing nanowires to control the neural signals and guide the cells for polarization will be useful for engineering complex architecture as well as the retina.

Acknowledgements

This research was supported by the Shinshu University, Nano Fusion Technology Research Group, Division of Frontier Fibers, Institute for Fiber Engineering (IFES), Interdisciplinary Cluster for Cutting Edge Research.

Competing interests

The authors declare no competing interests.

Author details

Davood Kharaghani[1], Zahra Tajbakhsh[2], Phan Duy Nam[1] and Ick Soo Kim[1*]

1 Nano Fusion Technology Research Group, Division of Frontier Fibers, Institute for Fiber Engineering (IFES), Interdisciplinary Cluster for Cutting Edge Research (ICCER), Shinshu University, Nagano, Japan

2 School of Optometry and Vision Science, University of New South Wales, Sydney, NSW, Australia

*Address all correspondence to: kim@shinshu-u.ac.jp

References

[1] Santos-Ferreira T, Llonch S, Borsch O, Postel K, Haas J, Ader M. Retinal transplantation of photoreceptors results in donor–host cytoplasmic exchange. Nature Communications. 2016;**7**:13028

[2] Patel BB, Sharma AD, Mammadova N, Sandquist EJ, Uz M, Mallapragada SK, et al. Nanoengineered biomaterials for retinal repair. In: Nanoengineered Biomaterials for Regenerative Medicine. Elsevier; 2019. pp. 215-264. DOI: 10.1016/B978-0-12-813355-2.00010-7

[3] Shang F. View of cellular biology through the eye. Current Molecular Medicine. 2017;**17**(4):247-248

[4] Kharaghani D, Khan MQ, Tamada Y, Ogasawara H, Inoue Y, Saito Y, et al. Fabrication of electrospun antibacterial PVA/Cs nanofibers loaded with CuNPs and AgNPs by an in-situ method. Polymer Testing. 2018;**72**:315-321

[5] Ullah S, Hashmi M, Khan MQ, Kharaghani D, Saito Y, Yamamoto T, et al. Silver sulfadiazine loaded zein nanofiber mats as a novel wound dressing. RSC Advances. 2019;**9**(1):268-277

[6] Khan MQ, Kharaghani D, Shahzad A, Saito Y, Yamamoto T, Ogasawara H, et al. Fabrication of antibacterial electrospun cellulose acetate/silver-sulfadiazine nanofibers composites for wound dressings applications. Polymer Testing. 2019;**74**:39-44

[7] Kharaghani D, Meskinfam M, Rezaeikanavi M, Balagholi S, Fazili N. Synthesis and characterization of hybrid nanocomposite via biomimetic method as an artificial cornea. Investigative Ophthalmology and Visual Science. 2015;**56**(7):5024-5024

[8] Kharaghani D, Meskinfam M, Bertoldi S, Imani R, Balagholi S, Rezaeikanavi M, et al. Biomimetic hybrid scaffolds for eye orbital bone tissue engineering. Investigative Ophthalmology and Visual Science. 2016;**57**(12):221-221

[9] Kim K-O, Akada Y, Kai W, Kim B-S, Kim I-S. Cells attachment property of PVA hydrogel nanofibers incorporating hyaluronic acid for tissue engineering. Journal of Biomaterials and Nanobiotechnology. 2011;**2**(04):353

[10] Wei K, Li Y, Kim KO, Nakagawa Y, Kim BS, Abe K, et al. Fabrication of nano-hydroxyapatite on electrospun silk fibroin nanofiber and their effects in osteoblastic behavior. Journal of Biomedical Materials Research Part A. 2011;**97**(3):272-280

[11] Khan MQ, Kharaghani D, Nishat N, Shahzad A, Yamamoto T, Inoue Y, et al. In vitro assessment of dual-network electrospun tubes from poly (1, 4 cyclohexane dimethylene isosorbide terephthalate)/PVA hydrogel for blood vessel application. Journal of Applied Polymer Science. 2019;**136**(12):47222

[12] Lee H, Xu G, Kharaghani D, Nishino M, Song KH, Lee JS, et al. Electrospun tri-layered zein/PVP-GO/zein nanofiber mats for providing biphasic drug release profiles. International Journal of Pharmaceutics. 2017;**531**(1):101-107

[13] Kharaghani D, Khan M, Shahzad A, Inoue Y, Yamamoto T, Rozet S, et al. Preparation and in vitro assessment of hierarchal organized antibacterial breath mask based on polyacrylonitrile/silver (PAN/AgNPs) nanofiber. Nanomaterials (Basel, Switzerland). 2018;**8**(7):461

[14] Khan MQ, Kharaghani D, Nishat N, Shahzad A, Hussain T, Khatri Z, et al. Preparation and characterizations of multifunctional PVA/ZnO nanofibers

composite membranes for surgical gown application. Journal of Materials Research and Technology. 2018;**8**(1): 1328-1334

[15] Jiang Z, Song Q, Tang M, Yang L, Cheng Y, Zhang M, et al. Enhanced migration of neural stem cells by microglia grown on a three-dimensional graphene scaffold. ACS Applied Materials and Interfaces. 2016;**8**(38): 25069-25077

[16] Biazar E, Baradaran-Rafii A, Heidari-keshel S, Tavakolifard S. Oriented nanofibrous silk as a natural scaffold for ocular epithelial regeneration. Journal of Biomaterials Science, Polymer Edition. 2015;**26**(16): 1139-1151

[17] Komez A, Baran ET, Erdem U, Hasirci N, Hasirci V. Construction of a patterned hydrogel—Fibrous mat bilayer structure to mimic choroid and Bruch's membrane layers of retina. Journal of Biomedical Materials Research Part A. 2016;**104**(9):2166-2177

[18] Shrestha BK, Shrestha S, Baral ER, Lee JY, Kim B-S, Park CH, et al. π-Conjugated polyaniline-assisted flexible titania nanotubes with controlled surface morphology as regenerative medicine in nerve cell growth. Chemical Engineering Journal. 2019;**360**:701-713

[19] Hunt NC, Hallam D, Karimi A, Mellough CB, Chen J, Steel DH, et al. 3D culture of human pluripotent stem cells in RGD-alginate hydrogel improves retinal tissue development. Acta Biomaterialia. 2017;**49**:329-343

[20] Xiang P, Wu K-C, Zhu Y, Xiang L, Li C, Chen D-L, et al. A novel Bruch's membrane-mimetic electrospun substrate scaffold for human retinal pigment epithelium cells. Biomaterials. 2014;**35**(37):9777-9788

[21] Chan SY, Chan BQY, Liu Z, Parikh BH, Zhang K, Lin Q, et al. Electrospun pectin-polyhydroxybutyrate nanofibers for retinal tissue engineering. ACS Omega. 2017;**2**(12):8959-8968

[22] Sun B, Zhou Z, Li D, Wu T, Zheng H, Liu J, et al. Polypyrrole-coated poly (l-lactic acid-co-ε-caprolactone)/ silk fibroin nanofibrous nerve guidance conduit induced nerve regeneration in rat. Materials Science and Engineering: C. 2019;**94**:190-199

[23] Mo X, Sun B, Wu T, Li D. Chapter 24: Electrospun nanofibers for tissue engineering. In: Ding B, Wang X, Yu J, editors. Electrospinning: Nanofabrication and Applications. William Andrew Publishing; 2019. pp. 719-734. DOI: 10.1016/B978-0-323-51270-1.00024-8

[24] Khan MQ, Kharaghani D, Nishat N, Ishikawa T, Ullah S, Lee H, et al. The development of nanofiber tubes based on nanocomposites of polyvinylpyrrolidone incorporated gold nanoparticles as scaffolds for neuroscience application in axons. Textile Research Journal. 2018; **89**(13):2713-2720. DOI: 10.1177/00405 17518801185

[25] Lee H, Kharaghani D, Kim IS. Mechanical force for fabricating nanofiber. In: Novel Aspects of Nanofibers. IntechOpen; 2018

[26] Yan L, Zhao B, Liu X, Li X, Zeng C, Shi H, et al. Aligned nanofibers from polypyrrole/graphene as electrodes for regeneration of optic nerve via electrical stimulation. ACS Applied Materials & Interfaces. 2016;**8**(11): 6834-6840

[27] Hällström W, Mårtensson T, Prinz C, Gustavsson P, Montelius L, Samuelson L, et al. Gallium phosphide nanowires as a substrate for cultured neurons. Nano Letters. 2007;**7**(10): 2960-2965

[28] Kotsakidis R, Meffin H, Ibbotson MR, Kameneva T. In vitro

assessment of the differences in retinal ganglion cell responses to intra-and extracellular electrical stimulation. Journal of Neural Engineering. 2018; **15**(4):046022

[29] Mafakheri E, Tahmasebi P, Ghanbari D. Application of artificial neural networks for prediction of coercivity of highly ordered cobalt nanowires synthesized by pulse electrodeposition. Measurement. 2012; **45**(6):1387-1395

[30] Kim Y-J, Yoo C-J, Lee U, Yoo Y-M. Cytotoxicity of gold nanorods and nanowires on cultivated neural precursor cells. Journal of Nanoscience and Nanotechnology. 2015;**15**(8): 5617-5623

[31] Bechara SL, Judson A, Popat KC. Template synthesized poly (ε-caprolactone) nanowire surfaces for neural tissue engineering. Biomaterials. 2010;**31**(13):3492-3501

[32] Suyatin DB, Wallman L, Thelin J, Prinz CN, Jörntell H, Samuelson L, et al. Nanowire-based electrode for acute in vivo neural recordings in the brain. PLoS ONE. 2013;**8**(2):e56673

[33] Gällentoft L, Pettersson LM, Danielsen N, Schouenborg J, Prinz CN, Linsmeier CE. Size-dependent long-term tissue response to biostable nanowires in the brain. Biomaterials. 2015;**42**:172-183

[34] Dvir T, Timko BP, Brigham MD, Naik SR, Karajanagi SS, Levy O, et al. Nanowired three-dimensional cardiac patches. Nature Nanotechnology. 2011; **6**(11):720

[35] Yang P, Yan H, Mao S, Russo R, Johnson J, Saykally R, et al. Controlled growth of ZnO nanowires and their optical properties. Advanced Functional Materials. 2002;**12**(5): 323-331

[36] Xu AM, Aalipour A, Leal-Ortiz S, Mekhdjian AH, Xie X, Dunn AR, et al. Quantification of nanowire penetration into living cells. Nature Communications. 2014;**5**:3613

[37] Jaggessar A, Mathew A, Wang H, Tesfamichael T, Yan C, Yarlagadda PK. Mechanical, bactericidal and osteogenic behaviours of hydrothermally synthesised TiO_2 nanowire arrays. Journal of the Mechanical Behavior of Biomedical Materials. 2018;**80**:311-319

[38] Lin H-I, Kuo S-W, Yen T-J, Lee OK. SiNWs biophysically regulate the fates of human mesenchymal stem cells. Scientific Reports. 2018;**8**(1):12913

[39] Li Z, Persson H, Adolfsson K, Oredsson S, Prinz CN. Morphology of living cells cultured on nanowire arrays with varying nanowire densities and diameters. Science China. Life Sciences. 2018;**61**(4):427-435

[40] Kanski JJ. Imaging techniques. In: Clinical Ophthalmology, A Systemic Approach. London: Butterworth–Heinemann; 2007. pp. 44-45

[41] Tian B, Zheng X, Kempa TJ, Fang Y, Yu N, Yu G, et al. Coaxial silicon nanowires as solar cells and nanoelectronic power sources. Nature. 2007;**449**(7164):885

[42] Young RW. Cell differentiation in the retina of the mouse. The Anatomical Record. 1985;**212**(2):199-205

[43] Strauss O. The retinal pigment epithelium in visual function. Physiological Reviews. 2005;**85**(3): 845-881

[44] Ishikawa H, Stein DM, Wollstein G, Beaton S, Fujimoto JG, Schuman JS. Macular segmentation with optical coherence tomography. Investigative Ophthalmology & Visual Science. 2005; **46**(6):2012-2017

[45] Hoon M, Okawa H, Della Santina L, Wong RO. Functional architecture of the retina: Development and disease. Progress in Retinal and Eye Research. 2014;**42**:44-84

[46] Krumpaszky HG, Klauss V. Epidemiology of blindness and eye disease. Ophthalmologica. 1996;**210**(1): 1-84

[47] Bird AC. Therapeutic targets in age-related macular disease. Journal of Clinical Investigation. 2010;**120**(9): 3033-3041

[48] Pierce EA. Pathways to photoreceptor cell death in inherited retinal degenerations. BioEssays. 2001; **23**(7):605-618

[49] Sivalingam E. Glaucoma: An overview. Journal of Ophthalmic Nursing & Technology. 1996;**15**(1):15-18

[50] Pappas TC, Wickramanyake WS, Jan E, Motamedi M, Brodwick M, Kotov NA. Nanoscale engineering of a cellular interface with semiconductor nanoparticle films for photoelectric stimulation of neurons. Nano Letters. 2007;7(2):513-519

[51] Forbes JM, Cooper ME. Mechanisms of diabetic complications. Physiological Reviews. 2013;**93**(1):137-188

[52] Dvir T, Timko BP, Kohane DS, Langer R. Nanotechnological strategies for engineering complex tissues. Nature Nanotechnology. 2011;**6**(1):13

[53] Redenti S, Tao S, Yang J, Gu P, Klassen H, Saigal S, et al. Retinal tissue engineering using mouse retinal progenitor cells and a novel biodegradable, thin-film poly (e-caprolactone) nanowire scaffold. Journal of Ocular Biology, Diseases, and Informatics. 2008;**1**(1):19-29

[54] Redenti S, Tao S, Saigal S, Gu P, Yang J, Klassen H, et al. Tissue engineering using mouse retinal progenitor cells and a novel biodegradable poly (e-caprolactone) nanofiber scaffold. Investigative Ophthalmology & Visual Science. 2008; **49**(13):4779-4779

[55] Christiansen A, Tao S, Smith M, Wnek G, Prause J, Young MJ, et al. Subretinal implantation of electrospun, short nanowire, and smooth poly (−caprolactone) scaffolds to the subretinal space of porcine eyes. Stem Cells International. 2012;**2012**:1-8

[56] Piret G, Perez M-T, Prinz CN. Neurite outgrowth and synaptophysin expression of postnatal CNS neurons on GaP nanowire arrays in long-term retinal cell culture. Biomaterials. 2013; **34**(4):875-887

[57] SanMartin A, Johansson F, Samuelson L, Prinz CN. Microarray analysis reveals moderate gene expression changes in cortical neural stem cells cultured on nanowire arrays. Journal of Nanoscience and Nanotechnology. 2014;**14**(7):4880-4885

[58] Hammarin G, Persson H, Dabkowska AP, Prinz CN. Enhanced laminin adsorption on nanowires compared to flat surfaces. Colloids and Surfaces B: Biointerfaces. 2014;**122**: 85-89

[59] Wang R, Huang X, Liu G, Wang W, Dong F, Li Z. Fabrication and characterization of a parylene-based three-dimensional microelectrode array for use in retinal prosthesis. Journal of Microelectromechanical Systems. 2010; **19**(2):367-374

[60] Piret G, Perez M-T, Prinz CN. Substrate porosity induces phenotypic alterations in retinal cells cultured on silicon nanowires. RSC Advances. 2014; **4**(53):27888-27897

[61] Kang M, Lee H, Kang T, Kim B. Synthesis, properties, and biological

application of perfect crystal gold nanowires: A review. Journal of Materials Science and Technology. 2015; **31**(6):573-580

[62] Lee S, Jung SW, Ahn J, Yoo HJ, Oh S. Microelectrode array with integrated nanowire FET switches for high-resolution retinal prosthetic systems. Journal of Micromechanics and Microengineering. 2014;**24**(7):075018

[63] Pan YL, Noda T, Sasagawa K, Tokuda T, Ohta J. Sputtering condition optimization of sputtered IrOx and TiN stimulus electrodes for retinal prosthesis. IEEJ Transactions on Electrical and Electronic Engineering. 2013;**8**(3):310-312

[64] Stett A, Barth W, Weiss S, Haemmerle H, Zrenner E. Electrical multisite stimulation of the isolated chicken retina. Vision Research. 2000; **40**(13):1785-1795

[65] Gautam V, Rand D, Hanein Y, Narayan K. A polymer optoelectronic interface provides visual cues to a blind retina. Advanced Materials. 2014; **26**(11):1751-1756

[66] Loudin J, Simanovskii D, Vijayraghavan K, Sramek C, Butterwick A, Huie P, et al. Optoelectronic retinal prosthesis: System design and performance. Journal of Neural Engineering. 2007;**4**(1):S72

[67] Tang J, Qin N, Chong Y, Diao Y, Wang Z, Xue T, et al. Nanowire arrays restore vision in blind mice. Nature Communications. 2018;**9**(1):786

[68] Sealy C. Nanowires promise new ways to restore vision and movement. Materials Today. 2018;**20**:1-2

[69] Parameswaran R, Carvalho-de-Souza JL, Jiang Y, Burke MJ, Zimmerman JF, Koehler K, et al. Photoelectrochemical modulation of neuronal activity with free-standing coaxial silicon nanowires. Nature Nanotechnology. 2018;**13**(3):260

[70] Sommer F, Brandl F, Göpferich A. Ocular tissue engineering. In: Tissue Engineering. Springer; 2006. pp. 413-429. DOI: 10.1007/978-0-387-34133-0_27

[71] Theocharis AD, Skandalis SS, Gialeli C, Karamanos NK. Extracellular matrix structure. Advanced Drug Delivery Reviews. 2016;**97**:4-27

[72] Mouw JK, Ou G, Weaver VM. Extracellular matrix assembly: A multiscale deconstruction. Nature Reviews Molecular Cell Biology. 2014; **15**:771

[73] Varshney S, Hunter DD, Brunken WJ. Extracellular matrix components regulate cellular polarity and tissue structure in the developing and mature retina. Journal of Ophthalmic and Vision Research. 2015; **10**(3):329

[74] Halfter W, Sebag J, Cunningham ET. II.E. Vitreoretinal interface and inner limiting membrane. In: Vitreous. Springer; 2014. pp. 165-191. DOI: 10.1007/978-1-4939-1086-1_11

[75] Hollenberg MJ, Lea PJ. High resolution scanning electron microscopy of the retinal pigment epithelium and Bruch's layer. Investigative Ophthalmology & Visual Science. 1988; **29**(9):1380-1389

[76] Kharaghani D, Qamar Khan M, Kim IS. Application of nanofibers in ophthalmic tissue engineering. In: Barhoum A, Bechelany M, Makhlouf A. eds, Handbook of Nanofibers. Cham: Springer; 2019. pp. 649-664. DOI: 10.1007/978-3-319-53655-2_56

[77] Zhao L, Hu L, Huo K, Zhang Y, Wu Z, Chu PK. Mechanism of cell repellence on quasi-aligned nanowire

arrays on Ti alloy. Biomaterials. 2010; **31**(32):8341-8349

[78] Lee J, Chu BH, Chen K-H, Ren F, Lele TP. Randomly oriented, upright SiO_2 coated nanorods for reduced adhesion of mammalian cells. Biomaterials. 2009;**30**(27):4488-4493

[79] Lee J, Kang BS, Hicks B, Chancellor TF, Chu BH, Wang H-T, et al. The control of cell adhesion and viability by zinc oxide nanorods. Biomaterials. 2008;**29**(27):3743-3749

[80] Maya-Vetencourt JF, Ghezzi D, Antognazza MR, Colombo E, Mete M, Feyen P, et al. A fully organic retinal prosthesis restores vision in a rat model of degenerative blindness. Nature Materials. 2017;**16**(6):681

[81] Vodovnik L, Miklavčič D, Serša G. Modified cell proliferation due to electrical currents. Medical and Biological Engineering and Computing. 1992;**30**(4):CE21-CE28

[82] Prinz CN. Interactions between semiconductor nanowires and living cells. Journal of Physics: Condensed Matter. 2015;**27**(23):233103

[83] Shah S, Hines A, Zhou D, Greenberg RJ, Humayun MS, Weiland JD. Electrical properties of retinal–electrode interface. Journal of Neural Engineering. 2007;**4**(1):S24

[84] Lanzani G. Light touch. Nature Nanotechnology. 2018;**13**(3):181

[85] Garnett EC, Yang P. Silicon nanowire radial p–n junction solar cells. Journal of the American Chemical Society. 2008;**130**(29):9224-9225

[86] Gréget R, Nealon GL, Vileno B, Turek P, Mény C, Ott F, et al. Magnetic properties of gold nanoparticles: A room-temperature quantum effect. ChemPhysChem. 2012;**13**(13):3092-3097

Chapter 6

Hypoxic Preconditioning as a Strategy to Maintain the Regenerative Potential of Mesenchymal Stem Cells

Bushra Bashir, Mahmood S. Choudhery and Ijaz Hussain

Abstract

Mesenchymal stem cells (MSCs) are non-hematopoietic cells with high proliferative potential and multi-lineage differentiation capacity. MSCs are promising therapeutic candidates for cell-based therapies, and hundreds of clinical trials have been registered using these cells. Potential of stem cells is compromised with the factors such as disease condition and age of donor. Therefore, taking the cells from such patients for autologous use may compromise the benefits of cell-based therapies. It is therefore required to enhance the potential of these cells before use in stem cell-based therapies. Optimization of culture conditions is preferred strategies to enhance the regenerative potential of cells before use. This chapter briefly overviews the benefits of hypoxic preconditioning of stem cells to enhance the regenerative potential of cells in terms of their survival, proliferation, and differentiation.

Keywords: mesenchymal stem cells, hypoxic preconditioning, regenerative potentials

1. Introduction

Clinical use of stem cells is rapidly growing in recent years because of their capabilities to repair and regenerate tissues and organs of body [1]. Stem cells have self-renewal potential and can differentiate into cells of multiple lineages under appropriate conditions. They can secrete a large number of bioactive molecules that are involved in repair and regeneration of damaged tissues and organs. Based on their potential, stem cells are classified as totipotent, pluripotent, multipotent and unipotent. Fertilized eggs (zygote) are totipotent as they can make cells of all three lineages and extra embryonic tissue such as placenta. Embryonic stem cells (ESC) are derived from inner cell mass of 5 days old embryos and are pluripotent as they have potential to differentiate into all cells and tissues of the body except placenta. MSC are the most widely used cells and they can be isolated from various adult body tissues (bone marrow, adipose tissue, articular cartilage, synovium, synovial fluid, dental pulp, etc.) as well as from neonatal stem cell sources (cord blood, cord tissue, placenta) [2]. Currently, hundreds of clinical trials have been registered using MSCs (www.clinicaltrials.org) for various conditions such as degenerative brain disorders, stroke, cardiac dysfunctions, myocardial ischemia, renal disorders, wound healing, diabetes etc. [3]. MSCs exert their effect either by transdifferentiation into respective tissues and/or through their paracrine effects by releasing different cytokines and growth factors [4].

The potential of adult stem cells such as MSCs is severely compromised in vitro by culture conditions and by number of passages of the cells [5]. In addition, "disease conditions" and "age" of the donor also reduces regenerative functionality of MSCs and their clinical use for repair and regeneration of damaged and lost tissues [6]. It is pertinent to note that elderly population is the main portion of population for potential stem cell-based regenerative therapies. However, autologous use of cells from aged individuals seems not to provide the expected benefits of stem cell-based therapies due to age depleted function of stem cells from such patients [7]. It is therefore required to enhance the potential of stem cells before clinical use. Different strategies have been employed for this purpose such as growth factors preconditioning [8], mild heat shock [9], and glucose depletion [10].

Different pretreatment strategies have been employed to enhance the regenerative potential of stem cells, however; hypoxic preconditioning seems more effective for enhancing stem cell function because relatively low oxygen concentrations prevail in stem cells niches as compared to normoxic conditions. Hypoxia can be an effective strategy for enhancing the cells function because it can make the cells adapt external microenvironment, reduce oxidative stress, shift metabolism towards glycolysis, enhance proliferation, differentiation and maintain stemness, and improve their motility to tolerate the hypoxic preconditioning after transplantation [11].

2. Regenerative potential of stem cells is compromised with age

2.1 Effect of donor age on regenerative potential of stem cells

Autologous stem cell-based therapies seem promising for several diseases. As humans get older, stem cell function deteriorate like other cells of the body. Diseases, especially degenerative diseases generally affect elderly people and therefore using autologous cells for such patients may have practical concerns [12]. With aging, superoxide dismutase activity (SOD) declines [13]. Studies indicate that differentiation potential of stem cells is negatively related with age of donor [12, 14–16], and therefore cell potential to form osteoblasts [12, 15–17], cartilage [12, 14–16] and other cell types is compromised. Another important aspect for cell-based therapies, that is, proliferation is also adversely effected with increasing donor age. Choudhery et al. [15] indicated that the number of population doublings decreased while the time of population doublings increased for cells obtained from aged donors as compared to cells from the young donors. Similarly, number of the colony forming units, size of colonies and plating efficiency of aged cells decreases in vitro [13–17]. Overall, growth kinetics and differentiation potential of the cells are inversely proportion to the donor age [15–18].

2.2 Effect of in vitro passaging

Cell-based therapies require large number of cells to get the favorable results in patients. For this purpose cells are expanded in vitro before use in most of clinical applications [12]. Leonard Hayflick in 1960 described that after a limited number of cell divisions the cells stop dividing. Cell morphology changes and they become enlarged and irregular in shape. The cells undergo a replicative senescence and this limited life span of cells is called as Hayflick's limit [19]. In this way replicative senescence limits the therapeutic potential of stem cells. The differentiation potential of cells decreases with increasing number of in vitro passages. For example, bone marrow derived MSC showed decreased differentiation towards adipogenesis, osteogenesis and chondrogensis at late passages as compared to initial passages [20]. In addition, the proliferative potential of MSCs decreases after long term passages [21]. Human Wharton's jelly-derived mesenchymal stem cells showed significant decrease in growth kinetics and differentiation when cultured for longer time as compared to the cells in initial passages [22]. Feline adipose tissue derived MSC showed a progressive decrease in pluripotency and proliferation over continuous passaging [23].

3. Oxygen levels vary in tissues

The structural and functional microenvironment in tissues where stem cells reside is known as stem cell niche described for the first time by Schofield [24]. A cell niche maintains the identity and functional characteristics of resident cells [25]. Important identified stem cell niches are in bone marrow [26], vascular vessels [27], liver [28] adult kidneys [29] intestine [30] endometrium [31], oral tissue [32], skin [33] and adipose tissue [34]. **Table 1** shows variable oxygen concentrations in some important stem cell niches.

Organ/tissues	PO2 values	References
Lungs (tracheal, bronchial, bronchiolar and alveolar epithelial cells)	13–14%	[35]
Subcutaneous	3–8%	[36]
Adipose tissue	3–10%	[37, 38]
Heart	2–6%	[39]
Brain (superficial cortex to deep white matter)	3–5%	[40]
Brain (hypothalamus, hippocampus, midbrain)	0.5%	[40]
Liver (parenchyma)	4–7%	[41]
Kidney (renal cortex)	4–9.5%	[42]
Kidney (medulla)	2%	[42]
Pancreas (exocrine)	2.7–4.6%	[43]
Pancreas (endogenous beta cell)	5–6%	[43]
Stomach	6–10%	[44]
Small intestine Lumen Mucosa Serosa	2–5% 3–6% 5–9%	[45]
Large intestine lumen and mucosa Serosa	0–2% 4–6%	[46]
Uterus	2.5%	[47]
Bone marrow	1–7%	[48]
Umbilical vein and arteries	2.4–3.8%	[35]
Blood	5–13%	[35]

Table 1.
Oxygen levels in different tissue in-vivo.

It indicates that oxygen levels significantly vary in various tissues of the body and are significantly low as compared to normoxic oxygen concentration. Initially, oxygen level of 21% were adopted for in vitro culturing the cells based on normal oxygen conditions in environment, however, latter, it was realized that the cells grow better in vitro when cultured in those oxygen conditions which are representative of their respective niche.

Similarly, when cells are transplanted in the body, they face hypoxic in vivo environmental conditions [49, 50]. A large number of grafted cells die due to harsh in vivo environmental conditions (such as hypoxia) at transplanted site. The cell death due to hypoxic microenvironment is especially considerable for tissues that are not vascularized and or already injured or wounded [51].

4. How hypoxic preconditioning enhance stem cell function

4.1 Effect of hypoxia on gene transcription

The survival and functioning of stem cells in hypoxic environment depends upon their metabolic switch controlled by hypoxia inducible factors (HIFs). HIFs are transcription factors that are present in eukaryotes. They have two subunits, that is, alpha(α) and beta(β). Their α subunit has three isoforms (HIF1-3). The post translational modification of α subunit depends on hydroxylation which is oxygen dependent. When intracellular oxygen falls, α subunit forms a stable α/β dimer because hydroxylation did not occur. This dimer is transcriptionally active; it enters into the nucleus, binds to hypoxia response elements and initiates transcription of hypoxia sensitive genes [52, 53]. HIF3-α is the negative regulator of HIF1 and HIF2 (**Figure 1**).

Effect of hypoxia on HIF- α is different for different types of stem cells

GRP78-Akt axis induced by HIF1α is important in augmenting functions like proliferation and survival of MSCs under hypoxia [54].

4.2 Reactive oxygen species (ROS) and hypoxia

Reactive oxygen species are oxygen containing substances that are produced in cellular metabolism. They are detrimental to cellular functions. Hypoxic

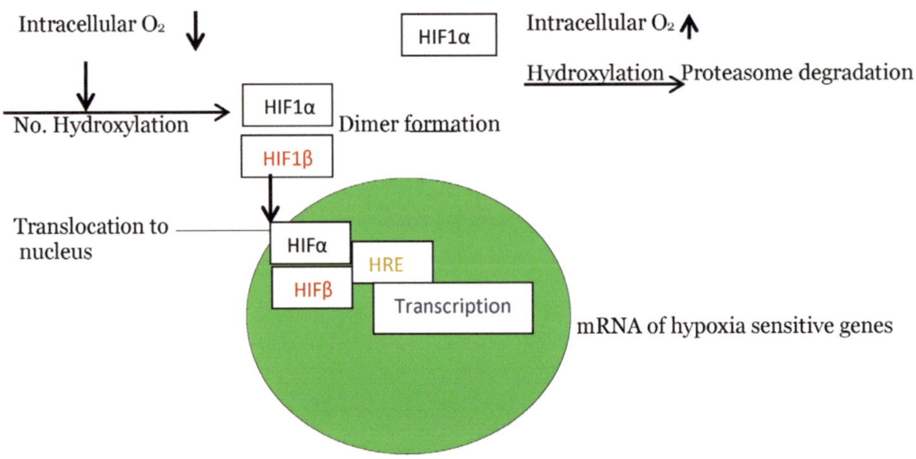

Figure 1.
Mechanism of HIF1 formation and transcription of hypoxia sensitive genes. HIF (hypoxia inducible factor), HRE (hypoxia response element).

preconditioning results in up regulation of Nuclear factor erythroid 2 related factor 2 (NRF2), which is a redox sensitive transcription factor involved in regulation of antioxidant genes [55]. Hypoxic preconditioning results in increased glycolytic metabolism and decreased tricarboxylic acid (TCA) cycle and oxidative phosphorylation. This mechanism leads to decreased mitochondrial ROS production and increase in the levels of antioxidant enzymes [52, 56]. Unbalanced redox homeostasis can cause stem cells aging and decreased proliferation. Hypoxic preconditioning augments redox metabolism [54] ROS acts paradoxically, at higher levels its cause's damage, and at lower levels it plays a role of signaling molecule. ROS also controls the hydroxylation of HIF1a, it causes inactivation of prolyl-hydroxylase enzymes (PHD), as a result degradation of alpha subunit does not occur and HIF1 formation occurs [57].

5. Hypoxic preconditioning improves regenerative potential of cells

5.1 Effect of hypoxia on stemness and survival of stem cells

Hypoxic preconditioning improves survival and stemness of cells and has been investigated in a number studies. SOX2, OCT4, NANOG and c-Myc are the markers that show stemness of cells. It has been found that stem cells grown in hypoxia are more viable, have decreased apoptosis through effects on HIF1a and p53 pathways [58].

When cultured under hypoxic (3 or 5% oxygen) condition for 5 days, stem cell markers were found to be statistically higher in dental pulp MSC [59].

PI3K/Akt signaling pathway get activated in cells exposed to hypoxia which in turn regulates many genes of cell cycle and CDK2 resulting in increased self-renewal and decreased apoptosis. Under hypoxic conditions cells switch their metabolism more towards glycolytic pathways and less towards oxidative phosphorylation resulting in less reactive oxygen species production (ROS) and more production of antioxidant enzymes [49, 60].

Hypoxia (1%) results in decreased senescence, increased lifespan of mesenchymal stem cells and were able to maintain proliferation rate, morphology and genetic stability [61]. Cryopreserved adipose derived stem cells cultured at 2 and 5% oxygen tension resulted in increased number and viability as compared to counterparts grown at 21% oxygen. In addition, all stemness related gene expression NANOG, SOX-2, REX-1, and OCT-4 were much higher in hypoxia group than in normoxia group. Another group demonstrated the upregulation of stemness related genes OCT4, SOX2 and NANOG in MSC grown in 3% oxygen culture conditions [62, 63]. Stemness of MSCs remains preserved in hypoxic cultures. Hypoxia results in decreased expression of apoptotic BCL-2 and CASP3 and increased expression of anti-apoptotic genes [64]. Stem cells derived from apical papilla of wisdom teeth also showed increased proliferation and upregulation of SSEA4 which is an embryonic stem cell marker surface antigen. Human umbilical cord derived MSC grown in a culture under 5% oxygen showed better proliferation and maintenance of stemness [65]. MSC derived from different sources showed increased expression of pluripotency markers Oct4, C-Myc and Nanog when cultured at 5% oxygen concentration levels [66]. Low oxygen tension also helped iPSCs from liver cells to preserve their stemness and decrease the time to switch from G1 phase to S phase, increase proliferation but the physiological oxygen level of tissue of origin should be kept in mind because these cells were grown in 10% oxygen level. The same group showed that culturing these cells at very low level result in loss of stemness [67].

5.2 Hypoxia improves differentiation potential of cells

Most of the studies use stem cells for regenerative purposes. MSC are multipotent cells that can differentiate into adipocytes, osteoblasts, chondrocytes and neurons under appropriate conditions [68]. The main advantage of stem cell therapy is living biological replacement rather than palliation through drugs. The use of stem cells to replace functional loss of specific tissue is determined by effective differentiation [69].

The results of differentiation are controversial; this variability may be due to:

1. Use of stem cells from different sources [70].

2. Due to heterogenous population of cells with similar morphology [71].

3. Designing of delivery system for successful transplantation of stem cells [72].

Biomaterials can be designed to act as carriers for the local delivery of stem cells, support cells or molecular niche cues [73]. Basal nutrients, cell density, spatial organization, mechanical forces, growth factors and cytokines have a profound influence on hMSC differentiation [71]. The role of hypoxia preconditioning in differentiation of stem cells into other lineages seems controversial due to inconsistent results of various studies [74]. Different studies have used different hypoxia percentages with variable times. Previously, cells were usually insulted with hypoxia using hydrogen peroxide, however, new trigas incubators have been developed recently that creates the precise hypoxic conditions even for longer period of times [59].

It has been shown that placenta derived MSC showed up regulation of osteogenic genes including osteopontin (OPN), osteocalcin (OCN), and alkaline phosphatase (ALP) as well as increased mineralization at 5% oxygen levels [75]. Another study found an increased osteogenic differentiation of human MSCs cultured at 5% oxygen for 5 days [66]. Contrary to this, multilineage differentiation potential including osteogenic differentiation of tendon derived MSc was compromised in hypoxia cultures [76]. Minsheng Yang and colleagues found that 9% hypoxia increased osteogenesis whereas 1% results in decreased osteogenic potentials due to upregulation of Notch 1 expression [77]. Cells cultured throughout in hypoxic culture (5%) showed less osteogenic potential, less mineralization as compared to cells primed with hypoxia (5% for 7 days). These results also emphasis that appropriate time for hypoxia is important to maneuver the different potentials [78].

Gale et al. analyzed the chondrogenic differentiation potential of equine synovial membrane and bone marrow derived MSCs and found no appreciable difference between cells cultured either at 5% oxygen or in normoxic conditions for 28 days. The results of expression of chondrogenic genes SOX9, ACAN, and COL2b were also variable between the groups [79]. Similar to this Li J and Pei M found no significant differences in chondrogenic index between normoxic and 5% hypoxic culturing for 7 days in synovium derived MSCs [80]. On the contrary adipose derived MSC showed better chondrogenesis and upregulation of several chondrogenic specific genes when grown in 2% oxygen cultures [81]. Bae et al. found increased expression of COL2A1, ACAN, and the transcription factor SOX9 in synovium derived MSC cultured at 5% oxygen levels. They also observed increased proteoglycan, glycosaminoglycans and collagen II contents from pellets in hypoxic condition [82]. Henrionnet et al. observed the effects of 5% oxygen conditions on bone marrow derived MSC cultures for their chongrogenic potential and resulted in efficient and strong overexpression of chondrogenic genes COL2A1, ACAN, SOX9, and COMP along with down regulation of osteogenic genes ALP, and RUNX2 [83].

Valorani et al. found that pre-exposure hypoxia of 2% oxygen level results in increased expression of adipogenic genes including peroxisome proliferator activated receptor γ (Pparγ), lipoprotein lipase (Lpl) and fatty acid binding protein 4 (Fabp4) and adipogenesis in MSC derived from murine adipose tissue [84]. Another research found enhanced adipogenesis of human adipose tissue mesenchymal stem-cell (hAT-MSC) exposed to 2% hypoxic conditions for 7 days before shifting to normoxia during differentiation [85]. 2% hypoxia resulted in increased adipogenic differentiation of dental pulp and periodontal ligament derived stem cells [86]. Choi JR et al. found decreased adipogenesis and decreased expression of adipogenic genes including LPL, PPARc and FABP4 under hypoxia (2%) as compared to normoxia cultures [87]. Another research also found a decreased differentiation of stem cells under hypoxia [88].

5.3 Effect of hypoxia on proliferative potential of cells

Hypoxic preconditioning results in enhanced proliferation and increased colony forming units as compared to mesenchymal stem cells cultured in normoxia. Higher oxygen tensions increase oxidative stress to cells and activate apoptosis [55]. Zhang et al. explored the effects of 1 and 5% oxygen culture conditions on rat bone marrow derived MSC and compared them with their counter parts at 18% oxygen level cultures. They found significant increase in proliferation along with upregulation of BCL2 (antiapoptotic gene) and down regulation of BAX (apoptotic gene) [89]. About 5% oxygen tension resulted in greater size, cell number and cell density of MSC colonies [90]. Antebi et al. evaluated the potential of cells at different oxygen concentrations and found that proliferative potentials of porcine MSC was higher at 1, 2, and 5% oxygen tensions as compared to normoxic conditions. They also found that 48 hour hypoxia in their study resulted in more proliferation as compared to proliferative potential of cells when cultured for longer times (10 days) [64]. Elabd et al. suggested that hypoxic preconditioning should be used as a strategy for in vitro expansion of MSC before their clinical use. They cultured human bone marrow MSCs in 5 and 20% oxygen and observed greater effects of hypoxia not on the regenerative potentials but also on the gene expressions of hypoxia exposed MSCs [91]. Notch2-c-Myc signaling cause's proliferation under hypoxia and inhibits apoptosis. Hypoxia can have a great effect on proliferation of MSCs [92]. Hypoxia (1%) increases the proliferation not only in early passages but also in late passages as compared to normoxic cultures and extends the lifespan of MSCs [61]. Significantly higher number of cells as well as increased viability of ADSC occurs in hypoxic conditions [93]. Rat bone marrow MSC cultured at 5% oxygen levels exhibited increased number of colonies and shorter population doubling time as compared to normoxic cultured cells [94]. Asadpoor Dezaki et al. showed increased expansion, population doublings, viability and colony forming unit fibroblasts in a group cultured in 2.5% oxygen tension than normoxia group [95].

Acknowledgements

I acknowledge the valuable suggestions and critical analysis of my colleagues at the King Edward Medical University, Lahore.

Acronyms and abbreviation

MSCs	mesenchymal stem cells
ESC	embryonic stem cells
iPSC	induced pluripotent stem cells
SOD	superoxide dismutase activity
HIFs	hypoxia inducible factors
HRE	hypoxia response element
ROS	reactive oxygen species
PHD	prolyl-hydroxylase enzymes
OPN	osteopontin
OCN	osteocalcin
ALP	alkaline phosphatase
Pparγ	peroxisome proliferator activated receptor γ
Lpl	lipoprotein lipase
Fabp4	fatty acid binding protein 4
NRF2	nuclear factor erythroid 2 related factor 2

Author details

Bushra Bashir[1]*, Mahmood S. Choudhery[2] and Ijaz Hussain[1]

1 Department of Dermatology Unit-I, KEMU, Pakistan

2 Tissue Engineering and Regenerative Medicine Laboratory, Department of Biomedical Sciences, King Edward Medical University, Lahore, Pakistan

*Address all correspondence to: bushra.b27@gmail.com

References

[1] Seetharaman R, Mahmood A, Kshatriya P, Patel D, Srivastava A. An overview on stem cells in tissue regeneration. Current Pharmaceutical Design. 2019;**25**(18):2086-2098

[2] George J, Manjusha WA, Jegan SR, Mahija SP, Josphin JS. A review of stem cells in regenerative medicine. International Journal of Scientific Research in Science and Technology. 2017;**8**(3):806-815

[3] Sousa BR, Parreira RC, Fonseca EA, Amaya MJ, Tonelli FM, Lacerda SM, et al. Human adult stem cells from diverse origins: An overview from multiparametric immunophenotyping to clinical applications. Cytometry Part A. 2014;**85**(1):43-77

[4] Fu Y, Karbaat L, Wu L, Leijten J, Both SK, Karperien M. Trophic effects of mesenchymal stem cells in tissue regeneration. Tissue Engineering Part B: Reviews. 2017;**23**(6):515-528

[5] Yang YH, Ogando CR, See CW, Chang TY, Barabino GA. Changes in phenotype and differentiation potential of human mesenchymal stem cells aging in vitro. Stem Cell Research & Therapy. 2018;**9**(1):131

[6] Neves J, Sousa-Victor P, Jasper H. Rejuvenating strategies for stem cell-based therapies in aging. Cell Stem Cell. 2017;**20**(2):161-175

[7] Brooks RW, Robbins PD. Treating age-related diseases with somatic stem cells. In: Exosomes, Stem Cells and MicroRNA. Cham: Springer; 2018. pp. 29-45

[8] Lu G, Ashraf M, Haider K. Insulin-like growth factor-1 preconditioning accentuates intrinsic survival mechanism in stem cells to resist ischemic injury by orchestrating protein kinase Cα–Erk1/2 activation. Antioxidants & Redox Signaling. 2012;**16**(3):217-227

[9] Choudhery M, Badowski M, Muise A, Harris D. Effect of mild heat stress on the proliferative and differentiative ability of human mesenchymal stromal cells. Cytotherapy. 2015;**17**(4):359-368

[10] Choudhery M, Khan M, Mahmood R, Mohsin S, Akhtar S, Ali F, et al. Mesenchymal stem cells conditioned with glucose depletion augments their ability to repair-infarcted myocardium. Journal of Cellular and Molecular Medicine. 2012;**16**(10):2518-2529

[11] Hu C, Li L. Preconditioning influences mesenchymal stem cell properties in vitro and in vivo. Journal of Cellular and Molecular Medicine. 2018;**22**(3):1428-1442

[12] Kretlow JD, Jin YQ, Liu W, Zhang WJ, Hong TH, Zhou G, et al. Donor age and cell passage affects differentiation potential of murine bone marrow-derived stem cells. BMC Cell Biology. 2008;**9**(1):60

[13] Stolzing A, Jones E, Mcgonagle D, Scutt A. Age-related changes in human bone marrow-derived mesenchymal stem cells: consequences for cell therapies. Mechanisms of Ageing and Development. 2008;**129**(3):163-173

[14] Lee J, Lee KS, Kim CL, Byeon JS, Gu NY, Cho IS, et al. Effect of donor age on the proliferation and multipotency of canine adipose-derived mesenchymal stem cells. Journal of Veterinary Science. 2017;**18**(2):141-148

[15] Choudhery MS, Badowski M, Muise A, Pierce J, Harris DT. Donor age negatively impacts adipose tissue-derived mesenchymal stem cell expansion and differentiation. Journal of Translational Medicine. 2014;**12**(1):8

[16] Gao P, Han P, Jiang D, Yang S, Cui Q, Li Z. Effects of the donor age on proliferation, senescence and osteogenic capacity of human urine-derived stem cells. Cytotechnology. 2017;**69**(5):751-763

[17] Zaim M, Karaman S, Cetin G, Isik S. Donor age and long-term culture affect differentiation and proliferation of human bone marrow mesenchymal stem cells. Annals of Hematology. 2012;**91**(8):1175-1186

[18] Zhang M, Wang Z, Zhao Y, Zhang L, Xu L, Cao L, et al. The effect of age on the regenerative potential of human eyelid adipose-derived stem cells. Stem Cells International. 2018;**2018**

[19] Wagner W, Horn P, Castoldi M, Diehlmann A, Bork S, Saffrich R, et al. Replicative senescence of mesenchymal stem cells: A continuous and organized process. PLoS One. 2008;**3**(5):e2213

[20] Banfi A, Muraglia A, Dozin B, Mastrogiacomo M, Cancedda R, Quarto R. Proliferation kinetics and differentiation potential of ex vivo expanded human bone marrow stromal cells: Implications for their use in cell therapy. Experimental Hematology. 2000;**28**(6):707-715

[21] Choi JS, Lee BJ, Park HY, Song JS, Shin SC, Lee JC, et al. Effects of donor age, long-term passage culture, and cryopreservation on tonsil-derived mesenchymal stem cells. Cellular Physiology and Biochemistry. 2015;**36**(1):85-99

[22] Rizal R, Widodo WS, Wibowo S, Munshy UZ. Effect of serial passage on growth kinetics, biological properties, and differentiation into adipocytes of human Wharton's jelly-derived mesenchymal stem Cells. Majalah Kedokteran Bandung. 2019;**51**(3):127-133

[23] Lee BY, Li Q, Song WJ, Chae HK, Kweon K, Ahn JO, et al. Altered properties of feline adipose-derived mesenchymal stem cells during continuous in vitro cultivation. The Journal of Veterinary Medical Science. 2018;**80**(6):930-938

[24] Schofield R. The relationship between the spleen colony-forming cell and the haemopoietic stem cell. Blood Cells. 1978;**4**(1-2):7-25

[25] Pennings S, Liu KJ, Qian H. The stem cell niche: Interactions between stem cells and their environment. Stem Cells International. 1 January 2018;**2018**

[26] Zhang J, Niu C, Ye L, Huang H, He X, Tong WG, et al. Identification of the haematopoietic stem cell niche and control of the niche size. Nature. 2003;**425**(6960):836-841

[27] Tang Z, Wang A, Yuan F, Yan Z, Liu B, Chu JS, et al. Differentiation of multipotent vascular stem cells contributes to vascular diseases. Nature Communications. 2012;**3**(1):1-3

[28] Kordes C, Häussinger D. Hepatic stem cell niches. The Journal of clinical investigation. 2013;**123**(5):1874-1880

[29] Ronconi E, Sagrinati C, Angelotti ML, Lazzeri E, Mazzinghi B, Ballerini L, et al. Regeneration of glomerular podocytes by human renal progenitors. Journal of the American Society of Nephrology. 2009;**20**(2):322-332

[30] Barker N, Van Es JH, Kuipers J, Kujala P, Van Den Born M, Cozijnsen M, et al. Identification of stem cells in small intestine and colon by marker gene Lgr5. Nature. 2007;**449**(7165):1003-1007

[31] Darzi S, Werkmeister JA, Deane JA, Gargett CE. Identification and characterization of human endometrial mesenchymal stem/stromal cells and their potential for cellular therapy. Stem Cells Translational Medicine. 2016;**5**(9):1127-1132

[32] Gorski B. Gingiva as a new and the most accessible source of mesenchymal stem cells from the oral cavity to be used in regenerative therapies. Postępy Higieny i Medycyny Doświadczalnej (Online). 2016;**70**:858-871

[33] Cotsarelis G, Sun TT, Lavker RM. Label-retaining cells reside in the bulge area of pilosebaceous unit: Implications for follicular stem cells, hair cycle, and skin carcinogenesis. Cell. 1990;**61**(7):1329-1337

[34] Berry R, Rodeheffer MS. Characterization of the adipocyte cellular lineage in vivo. Nature Cell Biology. 2013;**15**(3):302-308

[35] Keeley TP, Mann GE. Defining physiological normoxia for improved translation of cell physiology to animal models and humans. Physiological Reviews. 2019;**99**(1):161-234

[36] Spence VA, Walker WF. Measurement of oxygen tension in human skin. Medical & Biological Engineering. 1976;**14**(2):159-165

[37] Pittman RN. Oxygen gradients in the microcirculation. Acta Physiologica. 2011;**202**(3):311-322

[38] Saltzman DJ, Toth A, Tsai AG, Intaglietta M, Johnson PC. Oxygen tension distribution in postcapillary venules in resting skeletal muscle. American Journal of Physiology. Heart and Circulatory Physiology. 2003;**285**(5):H1980–H1985

[39] Rivera BK, Naidu SK, Subramanian K, Joseph M, Hou H, Khan N, et al. Real-time, in vivo determination of dynamic changes in lung and heart tissue oxygenation using EPR oximetry. In: Oxygen Transport to Tissue XXXVI. New York, NY: Springer; 2014. pp. 81-86

[40] Sakadžić S, Roussakis E, Yaseen MA, Mandeville ET, Srinivasan VJ, Arai K, et al. Cerebral blood oxygenation measurement based on oxygen-dependent quenching of phosphorescence. JoVE (Journal of Visualized Experiments). 2011;**51**:e1694

[41] Brooks AJ, Eastwood J, Beckingham IJ, Girling KJ. Liver tissue partial pressure of oxygen and carbon dioxide during partial hepatectomy. British Journal of Anaesthesia. 2004;**92**(5):735-737

[42] Zhang JL, Morrell G, Rusinek H, Warner L, Vivier PH, Cheung AK, et al. Measurement of renal tissue oxygenation with blood oxygen level-dependent MRI and oxygen transit modeling. American Journal of Physiology. Renal Physiology. 2014;**306**(6):F579–F587

[43] Carlsson PO, Palm F, Andersson A, Liss P. Markedly decreased oxygen tension in transplanted rat pancreatic islets irrespective of the implantation site. Diabetes. 2001;**50**(3):489-495

[44] Cooper GJ, Sherry KM, Thorpe JA. Changes in gastric tissue oxygenation during mobilisation for oesophageal replacement. European Journal of Cardio-Thoracic Surgery. 1995;**9**(3):158-159

[45] Korsbäck C, Höckerstedt K. Small bowel and liver pO2 during vasopressin infusion into the superior mesenteric artery. In: Annales chirurgiae et gynaecologiae. Vol. 73. No. 1. 1984. pp. 50-53

[46] Lind Due V, Bonde J, Kann T, Perner A. Extremely low oxygen tension in the rectal lumen of human subjects. Acta Anaesthesiologica Scandinavica. 2003;**47**(3):372

[47] Ottosen LD, Hindkjær J, Husth M, Petersen DE, Kirk J, Ingerslev HJ. Observations on intrauterine oxygen tension measured by fibre-optic microsensors.

Reproductive Biomedicine Online. 2006;**13**(3):380-385

[48] Spencer JA, Ferraro F, Roussakis E, Klein A, Wu J, Runnels JM, et al. Direct measurement of local oxygen concentration in the bone marrow of live animals. Nature. 2014;**508**(7495):269-273

[49] Abdelwahid E, Kalvelyte A, Stulpinas A, De Carvalho KA, Guarita-Souza LC, Foldes G. Stem cell death and survival in heart regeneration and repair. Apoptosis. 2016;**21**(3):252-268

[50] Krishnan R, Ko D, Tucker T, Opara E. Strategies to combat hypoxia in encapsulated islet transplantation. Surgery: Current Research. 2016;**6**:259

[51] Ezquer FE, Ezquer ME, Vicencio JM, Calligaris SD. Two complementary strategies to improve cell engraftment in mesenchymal stem cell-based therapy: Increasing transplanted cell resistance and increasing tissue receptivity. Cell Adhesion & Migration. 2017;**11**(1):110-119

[52] Lee HJ, Jung YH, Choi GE, Kim JS, Chae CW, Han HJ. Role of HIF1α regulatory factors in stem cells. International Journal of Stem Cells. 2019;**12**(1):8

[53] Suda T, Takubo K, Semenza GL. Metabolic regulation of hematopoietic stem cells in the hypoxic niche. Cell Stem Cell. 4 October 2011;**9**(4):298-310

[54] Lee JH, Yoon YM, Lee SH. Hypoxic preconditioning promotes the bioactivities of mesenchymal stem cells via the HIF-1α-GRP78-Akt axis. International Journal of Molecular Sciences. 2017;**18**(6):1320

[55] Dai X, Yan X, Wintergerst KA, Cai L, Keller BB, Tan Y. Nrf2: Redox and metabolic regulator of stem cell state and function. Trends in Molecular Medicine. 1 Feb 2020;**26**(2):185-200

[56] Salazar-Noratto GE, Luo G, Denoeud C, Padrona M, Moya A, Bensidhoum M, et al. Concise review: Understanding and leveraging cell metabolism to enhance mesenchymal stem cell transplantation survival in tissue engineering and regenerative medicine applications. Stem Cells. January 2020;**38**(1):22-33

[57] Cerychova R, Pavlinkova G. HIF-1, metabolism, and diabetes in the embryonic and adult heart. Frontiers in Endocrinology. 2018;**9**:460

[58] Lv B, Li F, Fang J, Xu L, Sun C, Han J, et al. Hypoxia inducible factor 1α promotes survival of mesenchymal stem cells under hypoxia. American Journal of Translational Research. 2017;**9**(3):1521

[59] Ahmed NE, Murakami M, Kaneko S, Nakashima M. The effects of hypoxia on the stemness properties of human dental pulp stem cells (DPSCs). Scientific Reports. 2016;**6**:35476

[60] Liu F, Huang X, Luo Z, He J, Haider F, Song C, et al. Hypoxia-activated PI3K/Akt inhibits oxidative stress via the regulation of reactive oxygen species in human dental pulp cells. Oxidative Medicine and Cellular Longevity. 9 January 2019;**2019**

[61] Lee CW, Kang D, Kim AK, Kim DY, Kim DI. Improvement of cell cycle lifespan and genetic damage susceptibility of human mesenchymal stem cells by hypoxic priming. International Journal of Stem Cells. 2018;**11**(1):61

[62] Safwani WK, Choi JR, Yong KW, Ting I, Adenan NA, Pingguan-Murphy B. Hypoxia enhances the viability, growth and chondrogenic potential of cryopreserved human

adipose-derived stem cells. Cryobiology. 2017;**75**:91-99

[63] Werle SB, Chagastelles P, Pranke P, Casagrande L. Hypoxia upregulates the expression of the pluripotency markers in the stem cells from human deciduous teeth. Clinical Oral Investigations. 2019;**23**(1):199-207

[64] Antebi B, Rodriguez LA, Walker KP, Asher AM, Kamucheka RM, Alvarado L, et al. Short-term physiological hypoxia potentiates the therapeutic function of mesenchymal stem cells. Stem Cell Research & Therapy. 2018;**9**(1):265

[65] Yustianingsih V, Sumarawati T, Putra A. Hypoxia enhances self-renewal properties and markers of mesenchymal stem cells. Universa Medicina. 2019;**38**(3):164-171

[66] Kwon SY, Chun SY, Ha YS, Kim DH, Kim J, Song PH, et al. Hypoxia enhances cell properties of human mesenchymal stem cells. Tissue Engineering and Regenerative Medicine. 2017;**14**(5):595-604

[67] Zhi X, Xiong J, Wang M, Zhang H, Huang G, Zhao J, et al. Physiological hypoxia enhances stemness preservation, proliferation, and bidifferentiation of induced hepatic stem cells. Oxidative Medicine and Cellular Longevity. 1 January 2018;**2018**

[68] Shende P, Gupta H, Gaud RS. Cytotherapy using stromal cells: Current and advance multi-treatment approaches. Biomedicine & Pharmacotherapy. 2018;**97**:38-44

[69] Hwang NS, Varghese S, Elisseeff J. Controlled differentiation of stem cells. Advanced Drug Delivery Reviews. 2008;**60**(2):199-214

[70] Rebelatto CK, Aguiar AM, Moretao MP, Senegaglia AC, Hansen P, Barchiki F, et al. Dissimilar differentiation of mesenchymal stem cells from bone marrow, umbilical cord blood, and adipose tissue. Experimental Biology and Medicine. 2008;**233**(7):901-913

[71] Pittenger MF, Mackay AM, Beck SC, Jaiswal RK, Douglas R, Mosca JD, et al. Multilineage potential of adult human mesenchymal stem cells. Science. 1999;**284**(5411):143-147

[72] Friedenstein AJ, Chailakhyan RK, Gerasimov UV. Bone marrow osteogenic stem cells: In vitro cultivation and transplantation in diffusion chambers. Cell Proliferation. 1987;**20**(3):263-272

[73] Lutolf MP, Gilbert PM, Blau HM. Designing materials to direct stem-cell fate. Nature. 2009;**462**(7272):433-441

[74] Wu R, Hu X, Wang JA. Concise review: Optimized strategies for stem cell-based therapy in myocardial repair: Clinical translatability and potential limitation. Stem Cells. 2018;**36**(4):482-500

[75] Camacho-Cardenosa M, Camacho-Cardenosa A, Timón R, Olcina G, Tomas-Carus P, Brazo-Sayavera J. Can hypoxic conditioning improve bone metabolism? a systematic review. International Journal of Environmental Research and Public Health. 2019;**16**(10):1799

[76] Yu Y, Lin L, Zhou Y, Lu X, Shao X, Lin C, et al. Effect of hypoxia on self-renewal capacity and differentiation in human tendon-derived stem cells. Medical Science Monitor: International Medical Journal of Experimental and Clinical Research. 2017;**23**:1334

[77] Yang M, Liu H, Wang Y, Wu G, Qiu S, Liu C, et al. Hypoxia reduces the osteogenic differentiation of peripheral blood mesenchymal stem cells by upregulating Notch-1 expression. Connective Tissue Research. 2019;**60**(6):583-596

[78] Inagaki Y, Akahane M, Shimizu T, Inoue K, Egawa T, Kira T, et al. Modifying oxygen tension affects bone marrow stromal cell osteogenesis for regenerative medicine. World Journal of Stem Cells. 26 July 2017;**9**(7):98

[79] Gale AL, Mammone RM, Dodson ME, Linardi RL, Ortved KF. The effect of hypoxia on chondrogenesis of equine synovial membrane-derived and bone marrow-derived mesenchymal stem cells. BMC Veterinary Research. 2019;**15**(1):201

[80] Li J, Pei M. Optimization of an in vitro three-dimensional microenvironment to reprogram synovium-derived stem cells for cartilage tissue engineering. Tissue Engineering Parts A. 2010;**17**(5-6):703-712

[81] Tabatabaei FS, Ai J. Mesenchymal endometrial stem/stromal cells for hard tissue engineering: A review of in vitro and in vivo evidence. Regenerative Medicine. 2017;**12**(8):983-995

[82] Bae HC, Park HJ, Wang SY, Yang HR, Lee MC, Han HS. Hypoxic condition enhances chondrogenesis in synovium-derived mesenchymal stem cells. Biomaterials Research. 2018;**22**(1):1-8

[83] Henrionnet C, Liang G, Roeder E, Dossot M, Wang H, Magdalou J, et al. Hypoxia for mesenchymal stem cell expansion and differentiation: The best way for enhancing TGFß-induced chondrogenesis and preventing calcifications in alginate beads. Tissue Engineering Parts A. 2017;**23**(17-18):913-922

[84] Valorani MG, Germani A, Otto WR, Harper L, Biddle A, Khoo CP, et al. Hypoxia increases Sca-1/CD44 co-expression in murine mesenchymal stem cells and enhances their adipogenic differentiation potential. Cell and Tissue Research. 2010;**341**(1):111-120

[85] Valorani MG, Montelatici E, Germani A, Biddle A, D'Alessandro D, Strollo R, et al. Pre-culturing human adipose tissue mesenchymal stem cells under hypoxia increases their adipogenic and osteogenic differentiation potentials. Cell Proliferation. 2012;**45**(3):225-238

[86] Zhou Y, Fan W, Xiao Y. The effect of hypoxia on the stemness and differentiation capacity of PDLC and DPC. BioMed Research International. 1 January 2014;**2014**:890675

[87] Choi JR, Pingguan-Murphy B, Abas WA, Azmi MA, Omar SZ, Chua KH, et al. Impact of low oxygen tension on stemness, proliferation and differentiation potential of human adipose-derived stem cells. Biochemical and Biophysical Research Communications. 2014;**448**(2):218-224

[88] Lin Q, Lee YJ, Yun Z. Differentiation arrest by hypoxia. The Journal of Biological Chemistry. 2006;**281**(41):30678-30683

[89] Zhang J, Xiong L, Tang W, Tang L, Wang B. Hypoxic culture enhances the expansion of rat bone marrow-derived mesenchymal stem cells via the regulatory pathways of cell division and apoptosis. In Vitro Cellular & Developmental Biology. Animal. 2018;**54**(9):666-676

[90] Caroti CM, Ahn H, Salazar HF, Joseph G, Sankar SB, Willett NJ, et al. A novel technique for accelerated culture of murine mesenchymal stem cells that allows for sustained multipotency. Scientific Reports. 2017;7(1):1-4

[91] Elabd C, Ichim TE, Miller K, Anneling A, Grinstein V, Vargas V, et al. Comparing atmospheric and hypoxic cultured mesenchymal stem cell transcriptome: Implication for stem cell therapies targeting intervertebral discs. Journal of Translational Medicine. 2018;**16**(1):222

[92] Sato Y, Mabuchi Y, Miyamoto K, Araki D, Niibe K, Houlihan DD, et al. Notch2 signaling regulates the proliferation of murine bone marrow-derived mesenchymal stem/stromal cells via c-Myc expression. PLoS One. 2016;**11**(11):e0165946

[93] Adolfsson E, Helenius G, Friberg Ö, Samano N, Frøbert O, Johansson K. Bone marrow-and adipose tissue-derived mesenchymal stem cells from donors with coronary artery disease; growth, yield, gene expression and the effect of oxygen concentration. Scandinavian Journal of Clinical and Laboratory Investigation. 2020;**18**:1-9

[94] Liu Y, Yang X, Maureira P, Falanga A, Marie V, Gauchotte G, et al. Permanently hypoxic cell culture yields rat bone marrow mesenchymal cells with higher therapeutic potential in the treatment of chronic myocardial infarction. Cellular Physiology and Biochemistry. 2017;**44**(3):1064-1077

[95] Asadpoor Dezaki Z, Kheirandish M. Hypoxia preconditioning promotes survival and clonogenic capacity of human umbilical cord blood mesenchymal stem cells. Iranian Journal of Blood and Cancer. 2018;**10**(2):43-49